Other Books by Fair Oaks Press

It's Not Your Fault

The 800-Cocaine Book of Drug and Alcohol Recovery

Aftershock

SURVIVING
ADOLESCENCE

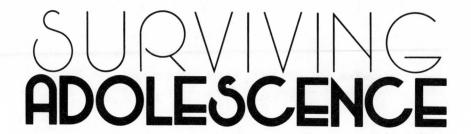

SURVIVING
ADOLESCENCE

HELPING
YOUR CHILD
THROUGH
THE STRUGGLE
TO ADULTHOOD

Larry Dumont, M.D.

VILLARD BOOKS   NEW YORK   1991

Library of Congress Cataloging-in-Publication Data

Dumont, Larry.
Surviving adolescence: helping your child through the struggle to adulthood/Larry Dumont.—1st ed.
   p.   cm.
Includes index.
ISBN 0-394-57405-2
1. Adolescent psychiatry—Popular works. 2. Biological adolescent psychiatry—Popular works. I. Title. 3. Parent — Child
RJ499.34.D86   1991
616.89'022—dc20   91-50066

Design by Levavi & Levavi, Inc.
Manufactured in the United States of America

9 8 7 6 5 4 3 2

First edition

Since all the permission cannot legibly appear on this page, they are begun here and continue on page vii.

Grateful acknowledgment is made to the following for permission to reprint previously published material:
   American Psychiatric Association: Criteria for Conduct Disorder, Separation-Anxiety Disorder and Borderline Personality Disorder, reprinted from Diagnostic and Statistical Manual of Mental Disorders, Third Edition, Revised, Washington, D.C., American Psychiatric Association, 1987.
   American Psychiatric Press, Inc.: Excerpts from "Cognitive Behavior Therapy with Children and Adolescents" by P. D. Trautman and M. J. Rotheram-Borus from American Psychiatric Press Review of Psychiatry, Vol. 7, 1988, pp. 584–607, edited by A. J. Frances and R. E. Hales. Copyright 1988 American Psychiatric Press, Inc. Excerpts from: "Adolescent Alcoholism and Substance Abuse" by R. L. Hendren from American Psychiatric Review of Psychiatry, Vol. 5, 1986, pp. 468–479, edited by A. J. Frances and R. E. Hales. Copyright 1986 by American Psychiatric Press, Inc.
   American Psychological Association: Excerpt adapted from "Impact of Adolescent Drug Use and Social Support on Problems of Young Adults: A Longitudinal Study" by Michael D. Newcomb and P. M. Bentler from Journal of Abnormal Psychology, Vol. 97, No. 1, 1988.
   Brunner/Mazel Publications: Excerpt from Beginning Child Psychology by Paul L. Adams, M.D., and Ivan Fras, M.D., Brunner/Mazel, 1988.

For those people in my extended family—Philip, Benjamin, Gene Prousnitzer, and Griffein and Danica Gould—to whom I offer a great deal of love, a wee bit of clinical insight, and enthusiastic encouragement to enjoy their teenage years.

ACKNOWLEDGEMENTS

The clinical staff I work with at Fair Oaks Hospital—Viola Sutherland, PhDD, Robin Shimel, ACSW, Queenie Vartoukian, ACSW, Dennis DeCicco, ACSW, Marlene Riordan, RN, Rose Christian, RN, Joseph Maglia, and Annette Hally.

To Andrew Slaby, MD, PhD, MPH, for his friendship and support.

To Lawrence Chilnick, for his encouragement in writing this book and his belief that I could do it.

To Karla Dougherty, who was invaluable in the preparation of this book.

Finally, I would like to thank all the young people I have ever worked with and hope that I have imparted as much to them as they have imparted to me.

CONTENTS

INTRODUCTION:
Our Teens Need Help

It is one of life's savage ironies that parents who tell their teenage children to enjoy these years as the best of their lives often recall their own adolescence with horror, shame, and embarrassment. As inevitable as puberty, emotional problems invariably appear during adolescence. The world was no better in the days of child labor than it was for teens growing up during World War II or in today's world with the threats of AIDS and substance abuse. The turmoil has always been there. Only the specific problems change.

But our perceptions form reality, and adults today perceive the world as a more difficult place for their children. In a recent survey by the National Association of Private Psychiatric Hospitals, 72.4 percent of all adults interviewed felt that teenagers today face far more serious problems than they themselves did when they were young. In fact, one third of the adults personally knew a teen who had tried to commit or actually had committed suicide.

As we move into the nineties, the problems of the past decade remain with us. The traditional family continues to disintegrate. Life-threatening drugs and activities are more accessible than ever before. Many of the rites of passage from puberty to adulthood no longer exist, and teens are maturing much faster than their parents and grandparents did. Children live at home longer because they can't afford to live on their own. AIDS has become a dangerous reality—despite the barrage of information on television screens and in magazines designed to limit transmission of the virus. Competition for entry-level jobs has become increasingly fierce. The cost of higher education has skyrocketed.

Here are some statistics:

- Suicide has increased 300 percent in the last thirty years among teens between fifteen and twenty-four years of age.
- There are 1 million teenage pregnancies each year.
- 77 percent of the deaths among fifteen- to twenty-four-year-olds are caused by accident, suicide, or homicide.
- Teens smoke and drink more than ever before.
- One million teens suffer from neglect or emotional or physical abuse.
- Between 3 percent and 5 percent of all teens have a learning disability and between 5 percent and 15 percent have a conduct disorder characterized by disruptive behavior.
- Only one thousand doctors in the United States are specialists in teenage medicine—leaving one doctor for every thirty thousand teens.
- Over 8 million teens are mentally troubled, but only 4 percent to 15 percent of them get the help they need.

Clearly our teens need help. Are they getting any?

A WORD ABOUT THE BOOK

Surviving Adolescence focuses on crucial childhood and adolescent development. It is my hope that by reading this book you will become familiar with the traits of normal adolescence, as well as the signs and symptoms of adolescent distress. Some of the findings might surprise you, some might provide informative insight, and some might even put your mind at ease.

I will explore specific disorders commonly found in teens—from eating disorders to anxiety disorders, from learning problems to substance abuse, from depression to suicidal behavior. For each problem you will find symptoms, unique characteristics, and reasons why they occur, which will help you recognize the disorder in your own teen.

The latter part of the book discusses the latest treatments and cures. Here you will learn about dynamic psychotherapy, behavioral therapy, pharmacotherapy, and more. You will learn when hospitalization might be required and how a hospital setting works. And, finally, you will discover preventive strategies that you, as parents, can adopt now, and you will learn how to create a supportive atmosphere at home and in school.

One technique we've had a great deal of success with is our Performance Group. By going out into the schools and the communities throughout New Jersey and performing skits in front of a group of their peers and authority figures, some of our adolescent patients have learned that their problems are not the end of the world. By sharing their pain with the various audiences, our patients have learned to trust others, to gain confidence in themselves, to be a valuable asset to others. They can conquer their problems, gain understanding, and make changes.

Solving problems in a positive way is the theme of this book. Through recognition and understanding, we can open the channels of communication between parent and child. We can offer help—and teens can accept it—in constructive ways. They can begin to take responsibility for themselves, to accept the reality of their—and their parents'—strengths and weaknesses, and eventually become healthy and mature adults.

You and your teen don't have to suffer. As a young boy I treated once said in a psychodrama session, "I have the confidence in myself that I can change and that the caring person inside will break through the barriers." The time has come to break through the barriers and raise the curtain on our myths and misconceptions of adolescence. The time has come to understand.

SURVIVING
ADOLESCENCE

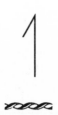

SETTING THE STAGE:
Infancy and Childhood

Birth is an astonishing miracle. When you first bring your baby home, it's hard to believe that this perfect little creature will grow up, that his hands and feet will lengthen, that he will begin to walk, speak his first words, and in a few years' time be going off to school.

The practical responsibilities of raising a child can easily become all-consuming—from learning to change a diaper to buying the right baby foods, from safeguarding your home to rating the best car seats and strollers. But giving your child a safe and healthy environment is only part of the story—and only part of the miracle of growth and development. An infant's body and mind evolve within an environment comprised of diverse biological, social, and psychological forces. These forces are responsible for the way your teenager appears today. Consider Brice, for example.

When Brice entered my office for the first time, I was struck with how poised and attractive she appeared. Here was a tall, slender fifteen-year-old girl with clear skin and a ready smile. Her clothes were in the latest style and she'd taken care to accessorize her skirt and blouse. She even shook my hand as she sat down.

It was hard to believe that Brice had tried to commit suicide on two occasions.

But a teen in pain can be an expert at disguise. In front of me, in black and white, were school records that revealed a grade level drop from "A" to "D." Here were her medical reports from the hospital when she'd tried to overdose on her mother's sleeping pills. Here were her family doctor's records that proved she was suffering from malnutrition.

Even without Brice's records, I would have seen the clues of her inner struggle: the way she avoided my eyes, the way she refused to answer my questions, the way she fidgeted in her seat after a few moments.

But after three sessions, we began to talk. I discovered that Brice was an intelligent, sensitive girl who had listened to her parents' battles for years—and who for years believed that she was somehow responsible for them. She had learned to avoid confrontation at all costs. She had learned to be a "good little girl" at school and at home in order to please her parents. When all of Brice's efforts came to nil and her parents told her they would be getting a divorce, Brice's self-destructive behavior began to emerge. It was the only way she knew to "lash out." She cut back on her eating. She lost interest in school. She dropped her friends. She became more and more insular, staying in her room with the stereo blaring. When Brice's father moved out, her mother also grew despondent; she herself was in so much pain that she had no room to help her daughter.

An extensive medical exam enabled me to rule out any physical disorders. Several sessions with her parents helped me determine that depression ran in Brice's family. And individual sessions with Brice showed me that the stress of her parents' divorce triggered her predisposition to depression. Brice needed to learn better ways to cope with her anger and with the difficulties of life. Some children are able to do this through psychotherapy alone. Some, like Brice, need medication as well as therapy to help them overcome a crippling emotional condition.

The medication I prescribed helped Brice alleviate her anxiety. After several months of both group and individual therapy, Brice learned self-awareness. And that self-awareness enabled her to discover less self-destructive coping skills. A year later, Brice has almost completely recovered. She has adjusted to her parents' divorce. She no longer feels responsible for their problems. She is positive about her future. Brice is one of the lucky ones. Her parents recognized the signs of struggle and did something about it. But sometimes it isn't so easy to see that something is wrong. And, as we will see later, sometimes what appears to be turmoil is in fact quite normal.

Brice's case is so complex—and compelling—because the development of a human being is a multifaceted "miracle." To understand this everyday miracle we must literally go back to the beginning. In this way the variables influencing the developing child come to be understood.

Your baby begins to develop physically and psychologically from the moment he or she is born. Nature and nurture—heredity and environment—complement each other, influencing your baby's development with every new step. Your child's environment triggers genetic predispositions, and heredity can influence his or her perceptions and responses to the environment.

One of my adolescent patients at Fair Oaks wrote:

Where is the child I once knew?
Let her out.
Let the girl show her face!
Don't keep her locked inside!
She is just destroying herself.
And soon, she will die.

To understand who your teenager is today, you too must go back to these early, dimly remembered days of infancy and childhood.

MASTERING A ROLE

A great story has a timeless quality: universal pathos and celebration combined with unique plot twists, motivation, and character development. A performance of a great drama will have the precision of a finely tuned watch—with the story elements working interdependently with the set, the lighting, and the actor's performance to create a mood and convey a message that ultimately gives way to critical interpretation. A developing child is like an actor in a great play.

In this chapter, I will briefly present the basic elements of child development—biological, social, and psychological factors—and major child development theories. By understanding how these elements interact, you will perhaps understand your child—and yourself—better. Sometimes living with a troubled teen can so dominate parents' lives that they lose sight of the many factors that combined (or conspired) to form their teenager. By taking a few moments to understand these key factors, parents will gain invaluable insights into their teens.

NATURE AND NURTURE: BIOLOGICAL AND PSYCHOLOGICAL FACTORS OF CHILDHOOD DEVELOPMENT

1. Genetics, Health, and Physical Growth

People truly are unique; except for identical twins, no two people have the same genetic makeup, and the permutations of new people are, according to psychiatrist Mary Chess, "greater than all the people who have ever lived on earth—even by conservative standards."

Even though our genetic patterns are all different, we still inherit our genes from our parents. Heredity, however, is not the only factor determining how a child will develop. Environment plays a role as well. Your baby's health depends not only on the genes he or she inherited from you, but also on the biochemical health of her uterine home. A mother who takes drugs, for example, is harming her child—regardless of the genetic makeup of the fetus.

Your infant's physical, psychological, and social growth intertwine and cannot be separated. To understand that toys can be held or put away on a shelf, a baby must be able to reach them. She must be able to turn her head and notice the toy on the shelf.

Physical growth continues throughout the childhood years. Hands and feet are the first to reach adult size. Faces start to mature as puberty draws near.

Height and width jump dramatically during middle childhood. We are all familiar with the small boy who sits in the front row during class picture time and a year later is standing in the back with the tall boys. On the other hand, we've also seen the number of girls who stand in the back in the fifth-grade picture, but end up somewhere in the middle row by the time sixth-grade class rolls around. Girls develop more body fat and wider hips as they reach adolescence, and usually stop growing tall, while boys develop more lean muscle tissue, which translates into strength, muscular bulk, and broad shoulders.

There are obvious differences between boys and girls—and the not so obvious ones. A study by Robert Hess and Teresa McDevitt at Stanford University found that girls and boys also differ in their reaction to parental discipline. Girls received negative scores on tests when authoritative appeals were made: "Why must you do it? Because I'm telling you to do it." But their scores were positive if explanations were given: "If you do this, it would really help me out. Can you think of other reasons why Mommy wants you to do it?"

Boys, on the other hand, had scores that remained the same—regardless of the style of appeal used.

This burst of physical development does not grow in isolated soil. Physical growth influences psychological and social makeup—in different ways for boys and girls. For example, a study done in California found that 56 percent of twelfth-grade girls and 43 percent of ninth-grade girls felt they were fat, but fewer than 25 percent of the boys did. The girls wanted to lose weight; the boys wanted to gain weight, size, and strength. (Incidentally, as proof that body fat accumulation and wider hips typify a girl's physical development, few of the girls were successful in their dieting.)

Girls may mature physically faster than boys by about two years, but mental growth does not always accompany physical growth. A girl or boy who looks older might be expected by parents, teachers, and other adults to act "grown-up"—a situation that can cause psychological problems. Ellen, a physically mature sixteen-year-old, was given more and more responsibility at home and at school because she looked "older" and seemed so mature. Unfortunately, the added responsibility weighed her down. Her teachers expected a more "serious" approach, while her boyfriend assumed her sexual behavior and attitude would match her physical development. She felt more and more pressure; she felt she had no control over her life. Ellen became depressed and dreamed of being "set free."

Boys who mature physically early are usually more muscular—which translates into athletic prowess and its resulting popularity and self-confident poise. On the other hand, late-blooming boys often have a hard time being accepted.

2. The Brain and the Central Nervous System

Besides determining what your child will look like, genes also program the size, number, and arrangement of the neurons in your infant's central nervous system. You might think the genetic pattern produced at birth would clearly affect the way your child behaves and responds to the environment. But, surprisingly, no study has been able to demonstrate this except in very extreme deviations. Genetics does, however, have a part in the way your child's brain develops. Here's how:

It seems the brain needs stimulation to develop fully. During childhood development, the environment provides the signals and the events that constitute that experience. But no one—infant or adult—can process all the information received from the "outside." Your child's brain must sift through all the countless stimuli in its environment and choose the ones to act on or store as memory. And your child's genetic predisposition will determine which stimuli to choose and which to ignore.

Your child's sex will also determine his or her brain development. Language skills are concentrated in the left hemisphere of the human brain. But girls have language skill involvement in the right hemisphere as well. Boys do not. Their right brain is primarily involved in visual-spatial relationships and abstract reasoning. Thus, girls are usually better at language than boys.

Boys, on the other hand, often have the advantage in visual-motor skills and mathematics, which use their right brain's spatial-relation and abstract-reasoning skills. When children first learn their multiplication tables, both sexes are equal. But when sophisticated algebra and geometry rear their heads, the boys usually shine. (Of course this is only a generalization and it certainly doesn't apply in every case.)

3. Hormones and Sexual Development

Hormones—sexual and others—regulate every one of our functions, from reproduction to physical responses to stress. They are the chemicals that enable the brain and the body to communicate with each other—through the brain-endocrine system.

Endocrine problems can be inherited and appear at birth or can lay dormant until they are triggered by environmental stressors (see chapter three).

However hormonal imbalances come about, the result translates into a body that does not operate at optimum level—and behavior that can seem extreme. Mood swings, anxiety, and cognitive problems can in many cases be traced back to endocrine abnormalities. For example, an overactive thyroid gland can result in symptoms of anxiety (shortened attention span, insomnia, weight loss, and hyperactivity) so severe that they closely resemble a panic attack.

The description of a teen with "raging hormones" is not far from fact. As your teen reaches puberty, there is a jump in both male and female sex hormone secretion by the pituitary gland. Estrogen levels rise in girls and its secretion becomes cyclic. Ovaries develop. Boys will also have an estrogen rise, but not as dramatic as their testosterone secretion, which results in testes development.

The primary culprit behind your teen's sudden need to borrow your razor and shaving cream is adrenal androgen, another sex hormone that increases its levels at puberty. Not only does adrenal androgen create the secondary sexual characteristics of pubic, facial, and body hair, but it also is responsible for the surge in oily secretions and adolescent pimples.

Don't forget your teen when it comes to visits to the doctor. Because adolescents are still developing, problems that might crop up when they are adults can be halted in their tracks. If there is a history of heart attacks in the family, a physician can encourage your teen to exercise and avoid saturated fats. He or she can be immunized against such potentially damaging diseases as polio, mumps, and German measles. Your family doctor can also help with birth control and avoiding sexually transmitted diseases. Further, he or she can see whether your teen is depressed and whether a weight loss or gain is the result of an eating disorder.

Some trouble spots for teens:

- *Eyes.* About one in four teenagers needs vision correction.
- *Hearing.* Loud music, especially through headphones, has impaired the hearing of millions.
- *Teeth.* Gum disease and tooth decay become increasingly common in the teenage years; almost half of adolescents develop a very bad bite.
- *Blood.* Since 8 percent of female adolescents and 3 percent of males have iron deficiency anemia, a hemoglobin or hematocrit test of blood is important.

Adapted from *The New York Times,* Personal Health column by Jane E. Brody, March 3, 1988.

The sex hormones might be responsible for the rise in a teenager's sex drive (and in many a parent's sleepless nights), but they are *not* responsible for your teen's sexual behavior.

Sexual behavior is more a combination of the social, psychological, and cognitive forces established in childhood. Though Freud called the years between early childhood and adolescence the latency period, it is not true that sexuality lies dormant. It might be less intense and less overt, but sexual issues remain part of a young child's life. A study of eleven-year-olds found that two thirds of them had felt they were in love and one half of them had kissed. The major difference between these eleven-year-olds and adolescents was that the majority of them believed that sex was something you did only to have babies. Not until adolescence do children discover that sex can be a sign of affection.

About 25 to 30 percent of young children will participate in homosexual play, but that usually has no effect on sexual orientation.

From infancy to age seven or eight, children will play indiscriminately with both boys and girls. From age eight to adolescence, they will gravitate to friends of the same sex—but there will be many late-night phone calls between friends about the opposite sex. At puberty, dating becomes socially acceptable and most kids will begin the dating game.

4. Motor Skills

Except for that first word, there is nothing that delights a parent more than a child's first step. Though a definite crowd-pleaser, walking— even at an early age—does not foreshadow a precocious intellect. Walking, along with crawling and sitting up, is locomotion—the use of the gross muscle system. Locomotion is one of the earliest motor skills a baby uses to explore the environment. He or she gradually progresses from using the muscles in the neck, chest, and shoulders to the muscles in the lower extremities. In their book *Principles and Practice of Child Psychiatry,* Drs. Stella Chess and Mahin Hassibi discuss a 1931 study that found five stages of motor development:

- Controlling the neck
- Sitting alone
- Crawling
- Standing
- Walking

One stage must follow the other—and all are connected to other areas of development. Controlling her neck means your baby can begin to perceive the world around her. Taking one step in front of the other means she can begin to walk alone—and learn independence.

At around twenty-four weeks, a baby will begin to use her hands and feet, scooping up toys and holding them, and gradually gaining control of her wrists and forearms. These are fine motor skills—which must develop before your child can learn to tie her shoes or brush her teeth. With fine motor skills, practice makes perfect. Children with highly developed fine motor skills could well be the artists of tomorrow; piano playing, drawing, and writing are all related to fine motor control.

5. Cognitive Skills

Cognition is mental exercise. It is how we think and gain knowledge. It is the mind wrestling with ideas and concepts, using the tools of perception, language, memory, reasoning, and judgment.

The three areas of cognitive development are perception, language, and conceptualization. Experience influences each one, at school, at play, and at home.

Perception
Children are not born with a preconceived view of the world. Perception is a gradual process, beginning with sight. As early as two days after birth, infants will show a definite preference for visual patterns—especially faces. Eventually, babies will learn to smile as a response to a familiar face, usually a smiling mom or dad.

Babies are born with their hearing intact. By eight months, they will show their interest in a particular sound by turning and looking for its source—a combination of motor and cognitive development.

Before your baby can move up to language, she must be able to hear, to distinguish different sounds, and to have enough brain development to store these sounds as memory. In fact, all her senses, from hearing to touch, must be intact in order for her to accurately perceive her world. And, in turn, her brain must be able to receive the information gathered from these senses—anything from a soothing lullaby to a cold, wet bed. This is called multiple-stimulus perception.

Language
There are two categories of language skills: receptive/comprehension skills and expressive skills. Receptive skills enable your child to under-

stand what is being said and expressive skills enable him to answer.

A child's new world of language is at first a mélange of different sounds: the conversations between mom and dad, the "baby talk" directed at the crib, the family dog, the vacuum cleaner, the musical mobile above her head. At first, children can only be receptive. They hear and understand only the overall tone of the message. Later they are able to pick up individual words.

By his fourth week, your baby will start to make sounds—and start down the path of expressive language. His ability to speak is connected not only to his motor development (his larynx, tongue, and jaw), but also his social development. He will begin to talk in front of others, and his new skill will be reinforced and rewarded by the amount of attention he receives in return.

By two years your child will discover that language is power, that it can make changes in her world. "No," for example, will almost always provoke a response from mom and dad. Your toddler is also developing his identity at this time—and as a way of expressing newfound independence, you might hear her say, "I hate you, Mommy!" Of course, she doesn't really hate you; she only wants to break away from depending upon her mother so she can discover more of the outside world.

Conceptualization

Until motor and perceptual skills have developed, your child cannot begin to conceptualize and solve problems. But as he learns to grasp objects, perceive what he is holding, remember his favorite bear, crawl and search it out on his toy shelf—as all this happens, he begins to be aware of the existence and the permanence of objects other than himself. He begins to see that there is a whole new world "out there," filled with guiding principles and patterns.

The key to cognitive development is interest—which is kept high through rewards and reinforcements. But in various studies, experts have found that competency is also a factor. A behavior is rewarding only when it exceeds a previously achieved level of competency. A child who has not yet said a word will be rewarded when she says, "Mommy." However, a "Mommy" from an adult will not get a round of applause. A child's interest will wane if he isn't challenged enough— or if he isn't yet developed enough to perform the skill.

Renowned psychologist Jean Piaget has contributed much of what we know about cognitive development, and I'll be discussing his theories later in this chapter.

6. Socialization

Human contact is crucial for all areas of development. It provides the rewards and reinforcement for brave new skills. It provides role models and learning by imitation. It helps create a sound, nourishing environment for healthy independence to take root and grow.

Socialization begins at home—with mother (or the primary caregiver). When a baby sees his mother's smile or hears her soothing voice, he will smile. In turn, his mother will smile back, and social interaction is born. Here, in rudimentary form, are the stages of socialization:

- From birth to one year, a baby learns to trust people. If the emotional attachment to the mother is balanced, if the child is neither too overprotected nor emotionally starved, and if basic needs are met, this sense of trust will flourish and the world will seem good.
- From one to six, a child will form relationships with people outside the immediate family, from nannies to other children, from relatives to friends of her parents.
- From seven to twelve, a child will become more independent. Friends and teachers become more important, but he will always identify with his parents on a deep level.

But socialization is not just a product of age. Parents must prepare their child for the outside world. They must show their daughter to use her knife and fork. They must teach their son to say "thank you." They must regulate sleep and provide toilet training.

Families themselves are complex and dynamic, and a child will have a relationship with each family member. By seven months, she will perceive her parents as two separate people with two very important roles. If she is an older sibling, she might take on a parental role, nurturing and disciplining her younger brother. She might also be jealous of him, viewing him as the "usurper to her throne." If she is a younger sibling, she might be treated like "the baby" and become overly dependent.

All these relationships influence each other. A crying baby, for instance, will influence the way his mother reacts to him—especially if he's been crying for hours. The parents' relationship with each other can also influence their child. A 1976 study found that happily married couples rewarded their children more and punished them less than unhappy couples. A child who receives positive feedback feels more confident and is usually more willing to ask for help (since he is not constantly criticized). The parents' relationship influences the children's self-esteem and views on marriage later in life.

A family's social class can also influence a child's social development. Studies have found that low-income families are depressed more often than higher-income families. Financial trouble, exhaustion, and stress all play a role in the way a family interacts.

Finally, there is the structure of the family itself. A new brother or sister, growing up, a move to another town, a divorce—all these things change the family structure and the socialization that is taking place. Successes and failures outside the home will also affect life within the family—and vice versa.

In the first few months of life socialization outside the family sphere is rare. Until a child is two or three years old, there is little interaction with peers. He will play by himself. If he has a "play date," he will still play solitary games, unless his friend takes his toy. Within the next few years, friendships will be made—but they will be based more on a common activity than companionship. But as a child approaches adolescence, she matures cognitively, socially, and emotionally. She begins to share feelings and ideas with friends. Deeper relationships are born— *if* her family environment first provided a stable and nurturing atmosphere.

7. Moral Development

Values are not inherited; they are taught. But parents can instill their morality in their child only if their behavior is consistent with what they teach. If they preach the Golden Rule but in actuality are stingy and bitter, a child will become confused. If they preach that "all men are created equal" but their behavior is prejudiced, a child won't believe what they say. If they preach honesty but lie, a child can become disillusioned with life.

At first, your child can only understand that she must "obey the rules" or get punished. But as she approaches adolescence, right and wrong become more abstract. Self-criticism and guilt take the place of "getting caught." These new, unpleasant feelings of guilt provide the fuel to act according to her moral principles. Self-incrimination provides self-control.

As with every other area of development, the ideal environment for moral development is stable and calm. Anxiety, hostility, and depression can lead to immoral actions. An anxious child might lie about his poor schoolwork because he can't tolerate disapproval. A lonely teen might steal an elaborate gift to buy the friendship of the "cool kids" in school. A hostile child may automatically assume he will be rejected by others, and just to make sure, he might break a window.

8. Emotional Development

Infants can't sit up in their cribs and ask you to please change their diapers because they are wet, cold, and uncomfortable. They can't say their stomachs hurt when they have a touch of the flu. They can't tell you how much they love the nursery wallpaper or that being held by Mom is the best thing in the world. They can't talk about their feelings, but they can communicate them by crying or smiling. They learn that crying will get a response and, more often than not, relief from that uncomfortable, wet feeling. Infants also learn that a smile will be returned, usually accompanied by a pleasurable hug.

Emotional development takes place in two ways: affectively and subjectively. Affective expressions of emotion are the temper tantrums, the laughter, the crying, and the smiles. Affective expressions are changed by age and socialization. For example, a seven-year-old knows that screaming and kicking will not be condoned.

Subjective emotional states are more complex. They are the deep reasons behind the affective expressions. They are the ways a child feels at any given time, based on her experiences, family life, physical health, and cognitive development.

A child may also develop feelings of anxiety or depression as a result of the kind of parenting he had. For example, one study of depressed mothers indicated that these mothers were less communicative, were more critical, and tended to overreact more to mildly stressful situations (such as a child's visit to the dentist) than nondepressed mothers. The authors of the study suggest that the depressed mother's reduced sense of self-esteem leads to a feeling of futility and ineffectiveness in helping a child overcome a problem, diminishing a child's sense of self-esteem and effectiveness.

As an infant grows up, nonverbal modes of communicating give way to verbal expressions. Instead of temper tantrums, a child can discuss her anger and frustration. In addition to tears, there can be explanations. She can describe her feelings in words because she has also developed cognitively.

With maturity come the more complicated emotions:

- When a child can understand the nature of pain, she can feel sympathy. When she understands the association between her painful experiences and the painful experiences of others, she can feel empathy.
- Fear won't show its face until a child can perceive and interpret a situation as threatening. A small baby doesn't know that fire is dangerous. He might cry at the heat's discomfort, but he won't be afraid. But once he cognitively realizes that the fire can harm him, he will know fear.
- Anxiety is a partner of fear, but it is more ambiguous. It is a response to an anticipated threat—one that may or may not happen. Some anxiety is normal, especially when a child begins her first steps toward independence and away from mother. Dr. Margaret Mahler calls this anxious time separation/individualization and I'll be discussing it later in this chapter.

9. Growth of Identity and Self

"Who am I?" is a question posed not only by adults. Even children sometimes wonder who they are and where they're going. But though we might feel like different people at different crossroads, our basic selfhood, that part of our personality that makes us feel unique, begins to develop in our mother's arms.

A child forms an identity by responding to the caregiver's attitudes and behavior. At first, this usually means a parent. She will learn by imitation, copying her mother's gestures or her father's phrases. Unfortunately, this process can be filled with roadblocks. By imitating a parent, a child learns the negative along with the positive—which can mean anything from a mother's low self-esteem to a father's habit of cursing. A child can also perceive a different role for herself than the one her parents want her to convey. A mother who prides herself on her ability to speak her mind might find herself with a child who is stubborn, willful, and destructive.

Parents are not only role models. They are also a "mirror" that can reflect an emerging positive self-image—or break it into tiny pieces. If parents are caring and demonstrative, firm and consistent, their love will bolster and enhance a child's sense that he is loved, that she is good.

If parents are depressed, angry, or inconsistent, they can make a child feel worthless.

A child's identity is constantly evolving during his early years. The more your child grows, the more the world opens up. Teachers, clergymen, other parents all become role models that will be incorporated in the identity your child will ultimately call his own.

This is how we all develop. Some of these factors are biological. Some are a product of psychological influence. But all of them, in a greater or lesser degree, are a combination of nature and nurture. Obviously, there are many other factors besides nature and nurture that help to define the type of person your child has become. In fact, for most parents, the following section is the most important.

TEMPERAMENT: THE WAY YOUR CHILD ACTS

Watch a group of children playing baseball. Each one up will hold the bat and try to hit the ball. Each player in the field will be ready to catch it in a mitt held up with pride. Each one of these kids knows the rules and they all seem motivated and involved in the game. But watch the game a little more closely. Some of the children will be more intense than others. Some will run a bit differently. Some will be more moody, and some will pay a bit more attention to the game while others let their minds wander.

This phenomenon is temperament, a term used to define the way a person acts in a given situation. Temperament was brought into the developmental picture by Drs. Chess and Thomas, who showed that:

1. There is no direct one-on-one correlation between environment and psychological development.
2. Individual differences in child behavior can be noted in the first few weeks after birth.
3. Mothers are not totally responsible for a child's mental disorder.
4. The temperament of a child will influence development.

By observing and measuring a child's activity level and his adaptability, her intensity of mood and his attention span, Drs. Chess and Thomas came up with three major categories of temperance that will influence your child's development and behavior: the Difficult Child, the Easy Child, and the Slow-to-Warm-Up Child. Let's briefly go over them now.

The Difficult Child

The difficult child is what he seems: moody, intense, withdrawn, and slow to adapt to new situations. During his infancy, he will be biologically irregular—waking up in the middle of the night, crying, refusing to eat, and wetting his diaper right after it has been changed. Unfortunately, this behavior gives parents many sleepless days and nights—and might, in turn, give the child negative feedback. His parents begin to feel responsible for their baby's wayward behavior; they lose confidence in their ability to raise him. But the difficult child does not necessarily have problems in development. He might require more patience and understanding, but once he becomes familiar with a new experience, he will show great enthusiasm and delight.

The Easy Child

The easy child is everything parents hope for in their new baby. She is predictable and regular in her sleep and eating patterns. Her mood is bright and she is eager to approach new situations. She adapts readily to change. Obviously, child-rearing goes smoothly with the easy child and parents feel justifiably rewarded for their love.

The Slow-to-Warm-Up Child

The slow-to-warm-up child is the shy child—the girl who hides behind her mother's skirts when she meets a strange new friend, the boy who withdraws from the group to play by himself in the corner. At first glance, this child seems anxious, but, in reality, she is a patient observer who, over time, will join in. Rather than exuberance, she will relish quiet enjoyment.

In addition to influencing the way a child acts, temperament influences development via a secondary route. It affects the way a child's parents raise her and react to her and the way the child copes with the stresses of life. It will help shape her attitudes and values. And it can make her vulnerable to mental disorders as she grows up.

Childhood development encompasses a wide range of influential biological and sociological factors. Is it surprising, then, that a diverse number of theories have arisen to explain this development?

MAJOR THEORIES OF CHILDHOOD DEVELOPMENT

Picture a little girl named Jenny, born just a few weeks ago. All she does is gurgle and sleep. But as time progresses, she develops use of her muscles and begins to perceive a glorious new world. Concurrently, she becomes aware of the comfort and safety of her mother's embrace. In a few years Jenny becomes a toddler. She exerts her independence by crawling away from mom, but she is soon drawn back to mom's security. She frequently chooses dad over mom and enjoys the pleasure and the power she receives by talking. She has play dates and playmates and she can dress herself. Eventually, Jenny goes off to school and she spends less and less time with mom and dad. Her friends, her schoolwork, and her burgeoning self take center stage. Jenny is on her way to puberty and another new world to meet.

This sparse scenario can be interpreted many different ways. Childhood development theorists have explored and explained the phases of childhood development—and the *why* of both normal and troubled youth. Though each of these brilliant minds has come up with its own theory, all the theories are pieces of the same puzzle. Taken together, they create a whole that is greater than its parts. They help us go back to a teenager's roots and discover where problems might have begun. Here is an overview of a few of the theories that have molded modern child psychiatry:

1. Sigmund Freud's Intrapsychic Conflict

Freud believed that conflict is a fact of life, and that the conflict between our instinctual drives and society's dictates creates our personality. Because immediate gratification of our instinctual drives is not compatible with the norms of society, we must learn to compromise and find more acceptable ways of satisfaction.

Take Jenny. As an infant, her instinctual needs are met almost immediately. She sleeps when she is tired; she eats when she is hungry. But as she grows up, she is faced with reality. Needs are not always gratified immediately. She learns to speak and think. Her conscious mind takes over, controlling her activities and behavior. She uses her cognitive skills to find an acceptable and positive way to control her more primitive and instinctual desires.

Nowhere is this seen more than in Freud's psychosexual development theory. In his oral phase, a child has no knowledge of the difference between his own desires and reality. He is completely narcissistic. As he begins to develop, the child moves on to the anal phase—which coincides with toilet training and a preoccupation with elimination. Here, the child has begun to think and is learning to perceive society's reality. Finally, the child moves on to the phallic phase. During this period, boys become enamored with their mothers and girls with their fathers. The defenses of the conscious mind, fear of retaliation from the same-sex parent, and reality awareness ultimately resolves this Oedipal conflict. The child will now identify with the same-sex parent—and receive instinctual gratification.

Freud considered the parent-child relationship the prototype for all future relationships. In fact, he believed that the neuroses experienced by an adult could be directly traced back to that person's psychosexual development. A child who doesn't move beyond the oral phase might become a dependent and self-centered adult. Fixation in the anal phase can result in a preoccupation with cleanliness and material objects. An inability to resolve the conflicts of the phallic phase can result in strained adult relationships and an inordinate amount of ambiguous guilt.

2. Anna Freud's Ego Psychology

Anna Freud took her father's theory one step further, seeing the conscious mind, or ego, as a separate structure independent of the instinctual drives. She believed a child is born with the capabilities of sensory perception and memory, and that these will develop despite a child's environment. But language, motor skills, and problem solving are developed only through the interpsychic conflict between the instinctual drives and reality. This conflict gives birth to the defensive mechanisms we all use—from rationalization to repression—to neutralize and channel our instinctual drives.

3. Margaret S. Mahler's Separation and Individuation

When Jenny was born, she had no concept of her existence as a separate entity. She was one with her mother and, to her, the feelings of hunger she experienced came from the same source as her mother's breast. Gradually, as she developed rudimentary motor and perception skills, she was able to see herself as separate from her mother. She might have pulled at her mother's hair or pulled her head away to get a better look at mom and the background environment. Dr. Mahler calls this the separation/individuation phase of development, and it occurs between five and thirty months.

During this period, Jenny began to function by herself. As separation from mom continued, she became interested in strangers—but only if mom was nearby. Exploration of her brave new world was still tentative, and her mother's approval and reassurance were needed to keep her on the path of individuation. If she had been blocked at this stage, Jenny might have found herself at thirty-five still needing her mother's approval, calling her when she bought a new dress or when she had to make a business decision.

The rapprochement phase occurs between sixteen and twenty-five months. As Jenny became more and more aware that she was separate from her mother, she also began to realize that her own wants and needs could be separate too. But the idea that her desires could be different from her mother's brought in a new variable: anxiety.

Anxiety is normal for all children during the rapprochement phase. Becoming a separate individual is a lonely task. A child can feel pulled in two directions: needing to run to her mother's arms and, at the same time, wanting to explore the exciting new environment her separateness has created. Learning how to cope with this normal anxiety is crucial for normal development—and coping can take many forms. One child might find the courage to dart away from mom at the playground—but she will turn her head to make sure mom is watching. Another child might focus his attention on other children or adults. And still another might occupy himself with various games in which he fantasizes his mother's presence.

This is a delicate time and it requires balance on the mother's part. If Jenny's mother was not watching her as she ran across the playground, Jenny would have felt both unwanted and terrified as she turned to look back. Her sense of self could have remained inadequate and she could have developed disorders later in life. On the other hand, if Jenny's mother had not let her run across the playground in the first place, Jenny would have grown up overprotected. She would have learned to cling to her mother, which would have ultimately created additional anxiety. Her need to sprout wings is an instinctive component of normal development, and it remains strong.

4. Erik Erikson's Interpersonal Stages of Man

To Erik Erikson, society and psychological development are forever linked. He believed that society influences each stage of an individual's development. For a person to adapt to his environment and feel secure, he must feel a sense of belonging. Further, as people grow, so do their interactions with society. Dr. Erikson saw eight major turning points in a person's life, from infancy to old age, where adaptation between an individual and society occurs. Each step can advance development or create roadblocks. The step below provides the fuel for the one above. Here, very briefly, are the four steps leading to adolescence:

- *Basic trust versus mistrust.* In this stage an infant is totally dependent on his parents. A parent's consistency and acceptance at this time are crucial if a baby is to develop feelings of self-acceptance and trust.
- *Autonomy versus shame and doubt.* In this stage, a child is beginning to move around his environment. He is exploring his world and beginning to control his biological functions. The responses he receives from his environment can either reinforce his newfound independence—or paralyze him.
- *Initiative versus guilt.* Here a child's cognitive growth enables her to express her wants and needs. If her family provides limits that are protective and supportive, the child will initiate interaction with others and gladly take on responsibility. But if her family is excessively strict, they will inhibit her assertiveness, and she will fear added responsibility.
- *Industry versus inferiority.* At six or seven years of age, a child is focused on learning. Mastering his new skills will foster his feelings of self-esteem and capability. Failure will make him feel incompetent.

The next stage, identity versus role confusion, occurs at puberty—and I will be discussing the adolescent's search for identity in the next chapter.

5. Jean Piaget's Cognitive Steps

In the pursuit of reason, Jean Piaget's theory of cognitive development stands alone. He believed that cognitive ability is developed in steps. Motor and sensory skills must be mastered before a child can successfully solve problems. And that mastery depends on the interaction between nature and nurture: the child's biological capabilities and his response to the stimulus he receives in the outside world.

Jean Piaget once gave his one-and-a-half-year-old daughter Lucienne a matchbox. Inside was a gold chain. The first few times, Dr. Piaget gave her the box half opened. Lucienne could see the chain and, through trial and error, wiggled it out of the box. But one day, he gave her the box only opened with a very small slit. Lucienne could not juggle the chain out; she couldn't stick her finger into the box. The opening was too small. She paused for a moment and looked closely at the box. She opened and shut her mouth. Suddenly, without the slightest hesitation, she pulled the box open with her finger. Lucienne had just graduated from the sensorimotor period to concrete operations.

Piaget's first step on the road to cognitive maturity is sensorimotor development—which lasts until a child is approximately two years old. Here, Jenny had just begun to interact with the outside world and just become aware that objects have different properties. Because imagination and thought had not yet been developed, Jenny would use trial and error to solve problems. She would keep trying to put a smashed toy back together again—without success.

Next comes the development of concrete operations. This period lasts from ages two to eleven. In the beginning of concrete operational thought, a toddler is egocentric. He believes that his is the only point of view in the world. There is no logic or cause and effect. Magic abounds. Stones can talk. Toys can dance. Reason is based on perception alone. When she squashed a clay pillar into a pancake, Jenny believed that the clay pancake was a brand-new piece of clay.

Eventually, a child learns to speak. He begins to express his feelings. He starts to understand right from wrong. Cognitively, he begins to realize that objects retain certain properties, regardless of what he sees.

Finally, a child develops the ability to do formal operations around the age of puberty. He can now understand abstract reality and is free to conceive of possibilities. His world of adolescence has begun.

Each of these theories has a different focus. Sigmund Freud saw conflict as the driving force in our psychosexual development. Anna Freud separated the conscious mind from our base instincts. Margaret Mahler focused on individuation and sense of self. Erik Erikson emphasized the interaction/interpersonal. Piaget concentrated on cognitive skills. Yet all of these different theories have stages that interconnect. Sigmund Freud's psychosexual development coincides with Erik Erikson's interpersonal stages and Margaret Mahler's separation and individuation phases. Combined, they provide a comprehensive and holistic view of childhood development.

But there's more. Early childhood development is not just the roots of a teenager's behavior today. *It is actually repeated during adolescence.* The steps a teen takes on the road to independence and maturity are the same ones he took as a baby. A search for identity. Exploring new worlds. Separating from one's parents. Learning new skills. Even a teenager's body begins a new developmental surge.

What was played out in the early parent-child relationship years ago is played out again—but this time, it is with both the family and the outside world.

Let us now leave childhood behind, jump ahead to those teenage years, and see, to the extent we can, exactly how and why teenagers act the way they do. One stage has ended, but the next has only just begun.

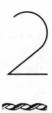

"WHAT'S THE MATTER WITH KIDS TODAY?":
The Adolescent Years

The prom was drawing near and Ruth had not yet bought a dress. She had narrowed it down to a red strapless and a print sheath, but she couldn't decide which one she liked best. She deliberated and deliberated; the decision was becoming as crucial as determining world peace. She finally asked her mother which one she liked best. Her mother picked the print. Ruth agreed and thanked her mom. The next day she went out and bought the red strapless.

Billy had been an "A" student throughout junior high school. But when he hit tenth grade, he turned in his slide rule for sneakers. Suddenly, it was baseball in the spring, football in the winter, and basketball whenever he could find a court. His parents were getting concerned about his grades, but Billy was never around enough to ask about them.

Eileen was a considerate, sweet child. She always smiled and helped her parents with the chores. She was well-groomed and fastidious—until she turned thirteen. The first thing to go was the smile. It didn't go with her black clothes and punk jewelry. Next was the help around the house. When Eileen wasn't at school or visiting her friends, she was in her room blaring music or talking on the phone. When her parents calmly tried to talk to her, Eileen would scream, "You're always picking on me!"

At last, John got a date with the girl of his dreams. Unfortunately, he made his date for the same night as his parents' twenty-fifth anniversary party. He didn't bother to change his plans because he knew his parents would understand. This was the most important night of his life. But his parents didn't see it his way. John broke his date—reluctantly. He was astounded at his parent's "selfishness."

These scenes might sound familiar. They are a slice of adolescent drama that parents everywhere—and at every time—have experienced.

Four thousand years ago, in ancient Ur, a craftsman carved this warning in stone: "Our civilization is doomed if the unheard of actions of our younger generations are allowed to continue."

A thousand-odd years later, Socrates was so angered by Athens' youth that he felt compelled to write: "Children today are tyrants. They contradict their parents, gobble their food, and tyrannize their teachers."

Adolescent behavior went underground during the Middle Ages. Children were considered adults by the time they were seven and, if they were lucky to have survived plague, disease, and hazardous living conditions, they would be married by the time they reached thirteen.

But the rebirth of civilization in the Renaissance also included adult complaints about the young. In *The Winter's Tale,* Shakespeare had an actor say: "I would there were no age between ten and three-and-twenty, or that youth would sleep out the rest; for there is nothing in the between but getting wenches with child, wronging the ancientry, stealing, fighting. . . ."

The settings and the costumes have changed. But whether it be the Industrial Revolution or world war, a Norman Rockwell small-town culture or an inner-city street, adolescent behavior has always perplexed, annoyed, and even frightened parents. Today is no different. As the curtain rises on the teenage years, a whole surge of physical and emotional development emerges. Rather than the transition years between childhood and adulthood, adolescence is, as I mentioned in chapter one, a repeat performance of childhood development. New intellectual skills, new emotions, new social behavior, new body shapes and chemistry—all are simultaneously occurring within your child as he or she begins adolescence. And all these changes are happening not only within the intimate family environment, but outside in the world at large as well.

WHY TEENS ACT THE WAY THEY DO

As your child reaches puberty, it may seem as if a stranger has invaded your house. But what might seem erratic and bewildering can be a part of a very natural process. Erik Erikson said that the crucial task of adolescence was finding a sense of identity—and, more than any other factor, it is that emerging self that creates such seemingly unpredictable havoc at home. Your child will be testing out new roles and new identities to find one that fits. He will be discovering that he understands abstract thought—and will experiment with different ideologies. He will find that his parents are not the only people in the universe and will want to find significant others on his journey. He will begin to recognize emotions within himself and within others—and will control and articulate them to get a response. Ultimately, these actions will strengthen your teen's emerging self.

Unfortunately, this burgeoning self is vulnerable, especially if growth was blocked during childhood development, if there is a great deal of stress at home or at school, or if a child is genetically predisposed to have problems. Sometimes a teen cannot articulate his feelings. Sometimes she does not have a realistic perception of herself. And sometimes she doesn't believe she is as "perfect" as she should be, which creates low self-esteem.

But before you can determine if your teenager has problems, you first have to understand what's normal—and what isn't.

Though no teen is completely typical, there are several characteristics that make up normal teenage behavior. In his book *High Times/ Low Times: The Many Faces of Adolescent Depression,* Dr. John Meeks describes the several characteristics that make up normal teenage behavior. Though no adolescent is completely typical, you will find that each description holds some truth about teenagers. Let's go over them now:

1. "My Parents Treat Me Like a Child"

Cal used to chatter to his parents almost nonstop. Whether it was stories about his friends, his teachers, or the interesting and weird things he saw during the day, he always wanted to share them during dinner. But when he entered junior high, he would concentrate more on his plate than his voice. His mother would ask him how school was, and he would say fine. His father would ask about one of his friends, and Cal would shrug and say Tom's okay. When his father asked him to throw out the garbage, he would storm out—muttering that he had to do everything. When his mother suggested he wear a raincoat on rainy days or a sweater in September, he would tell her he's not a child, that she should stop telling him what to do.

But when Cal's parents decided to back off for a while, he became upset. One day at dinner, he asked them why they didn't ask him anything anymore. He was sure they didn't care.

Cal's performance is typical. He is struggling between wanting independence from his parents and needing their approval at the same time. Like Ruth with the prom dress choices, he wanted his parent's advice, but he resented them when they gave it.

As we have seen in chapter one, small children are completely dependent on their parents. Safety, nourishment, and self-esteem all stem from their mother's and father's love. But as they begin to develop, their desire to explore the universe outside their parents' arms becomes strong. Margaret Mahler's separation/individuation process begins— with its inherent anxiety. But just as children make peace with the delicate balance between exploration and mom's protection, they become adolescents—and the struggle begins anew. Suddenly, they find it embarrassing to need their parents. Only babies want their parents to tell them what to do. Only little kids care so much about mom and dad.

Adolescents want to feel grown-up—and that means independence from the very place where they had received so much security and self-esteem. It's no wonder that "flying the coop" is fraught with anxiety. Since teenagers have not yet felt the self-confidence that comes from independent experience, they are constantly being pushed and pulled between wanting to spread their wings and wanting to stay in the comfortable nest.

One way teens deal with this struggle is to knock their "godlike" parents off their pedestal a bit, using what Erik Erikson called straw men to give them that extra push. It stands to reason that if a child's universe is her parents, these parents become all-powerful and godlike to her. These feelings ultimately become internalized into her superego, or conscience. But this superego can be a fearful obstacle to growing up and becoming independent. As Dr. Meeks explains in his book, if these teens "externalize this superego by knocking their parents—the straw men—off their pedestal, they can have an easier time pulling away." Here's an example: Jaynie's mother had left the answering machine on for a few hours because she didn't want to talk to anyone.

When the phone rang, the message played that "no one was home right now." Jaynie queried her mother after the recording was finished: "How can you say no one is home when you are home? Isn't that a lie? Didn't you tell me never to lie?" The pedestal gets kicked a little bit, the adolescent feels better about spreading his wings, and his conscience is still intact and calm. It's not easy for parents to adjust to this attitude, especially when they've enjoyed and basked in godlike attention, but it is normal—and it is a part of a child's growing up and learning to be independent.

2. "You Gotta Have Friends"

Margaret had a new best friend almost every other week. Her mother would come home from work and there would be Margaret, giggling over diet sodas in the kitchen with her latest companion. Weekends were for "hanging out" with the gang and after school meant going to the mall to buy a new dress for the latest party. It was almost as if she were running for "Miss Popularity."

Teenage friendship is an outgrowth of that push/pull struggle between independence and dependence. Without her parents to give her self-esteem, Margaret has to go elsewhere—and that means to her friends. The love and confidence she used to get from her mom and dad she now finds with her peers, and this quickly replenishes the well of self-esteem.

It's a fact. Teens feel "cool" or popular or well-liked by the company they keep. Remember back to your teenage years: If the most popular kids in school liked you, you felt popular, too. If the coolest kids called you on the phone, you felt special.

But these friendships are often superficial and narcissistic, built more on style than substance. They are usually a "quick fix," fulfilling the need for self-esteem—but without internal depth. Consequently, especially among young teens, these friendships are transient, constantly formed and re-formed.

There's also safety in numbers. Teenage cliques and groups are a way of life. With their own language, dress code, rules, and fads, teenagers form a counterculture—a solid front to show their "superiority" over their parents and to hide, at least on the surface, their inner uncertainty. Rejection and acceptance become a daily way of life. Because they don't yet have a clear picture of themselves, teenagers will always be wondering if their friends really are as popular as they think they are. Maybe they're really nerds. Maybe those teens standing at the other end of the hall are hipper. . . . Ultimately, most teenage friendships will end as fast as they begin.

As teenagers continue to grow and mature, so do their friendships. As their real self-image develops inside, teens no longer have to look outside for approval. They become more comfortable with themselves. Friendships no longer are based on a "top ten" list of who's popular and cool. Teens begin to make real friends based on mutuality. They choose friends for who they are—not what they are.

3. "My Son Is Always on the Move"

Whether it was basketball practice after school, an all-nighter the day of the prom, a weekend camping trip with his friends, or cramming for a midterm test after delivering papers in the neighborhood, Billy was always going strong—and always with good cheer. He might be up almost half the night, but he'd still come to the breakfast table singing. In fact, he had so much energy, his parents got tired just looking at him.

WHAT DO TEENS WANT TO KNOW ABOUT SEX?

Here are some questions from *What Teenagers Want to Know About Sex: Questions and Answers* by Boston Children's Hospital:

- Once I've had intercourse, will I automatically want to sleep with the next person I like?
- What happens to the male's body if sperm are not released?
- Is there a male counterpart to menopause?
- Is it normal not to have menstrual cramps?
- Does a male ever have a "safe" period?
- If a female does not feel any sexual desire during intercourse, can she still get pregnant?
- If a female does not use birth control, what are her chances of getting pregnant?
- How can a person avoid getting a sexually transmitted disease?

Reprinted from *USA Today,* Health and Behavior column by Anita Manning, October 3, 1988.

Teens are active. Period. Their bodies are developing and they need to use their newfound muscles. In his studies of childhood development, Jean Piaget found that children will repeat a learned skill until it is mastered. Similarly, in adolescence, teens will use their newly developed fine motor skills and their increased voluntary muscle mass over and over again.

The burst of hormones that's surging through a developing teen's body is also responsible for that extra energy. The added estrogen, adrenaline, steroids, and testosterone chemically translate into energy. But physiology is only part of the action. There are psychological factors at work as well. To a teen, passivity equals that "awful" dependence—but action means independence. This attitude is fostered by adults. We don't usually ask teens about their thoughts or feelings. Instead, we'll ask goal-oriented questions: "What careers do you have in mind?" "Where do you want to go to college?" "Who are you going out with now?"

And, in fact, teens are supposed to be doing things. Society permits action and fosters independence. Your teen can do more things than he or she could ever have imagined as a child. Your son can pick you up at the commuter train station in the family car. Your daughter can buy her own clothes and personal items. Your son can date and work part-time. Your daughter no longer needs to ask your permission to cross the street.

4. "What You See Isn't Necessarily What You Get"

Christine loved to make an entrance. She'd come down the stairs to meet a blind date like a movie star meeting her fans. She appeared poised and elegant in the clothes she painstakingly handpicked during her hours at the mall. She smiled just like her favorite model in her favorite magazine. But Christine's aura was a façade. She might exude confidence, but inside she was terrified of being rejected.

Christopher, on the other hand, acted aloof and quiet when he went to a party. He'd tell his friends he didn't expect to meet anyone, and he presented the quintessential picture of someone with little confidence. It was a self-fulfilling prophecy for Chris: he didn't expect to meet anyone, and so he didn't.

Like actors looking for the part that will make their careers, teenagers are constantly trying on different roles. They are beginning to believe in their talents, but their abilities lag behind their expectations. They can see what they need for success, but they haven't yet tested their performance in the theater of life. Sometimes, a teen will see a stage full of bungling amateurs, just waiting for him to step in and take charge of the scene. But other times, a teen will see herself with little talent, surrounded by award-winning professionals. Suffering from stage fright, she won't even try out for a part.

Instead of showing their fear, some teens, like Christine, will give an aura of exaggerated confidence. Others, like Christopher, will wear their lack of confidence as a shield. If they act timid and quiet, they won't be expected to succeed. And, if in spite of themselves, they do get that date, they can chalk it up to luck.

This role-playing can make for stubborn streaks. Jaynie, for example, had an older sister who was a cheerleader. Jaynie saw how popular her sister was and she got it into her head that if she too became a cheerleader, the world would be hers for the asking. Unfortunately, Jaynie had two left feet and could never make the grade. But throughout high school, she kept trying and trying—and getting rejected.

5. "I Love You, Mom." "I Hate You, Mom!"

As Mary's mother told her neighbor over coffee, it was as if she had two teenage daughters, not just one. Her daughter Mary would wake up exuberant and chatty, eating breakfast and getting dressed while talking a mile a minute. That same night, Mary would be sullen. She'd barely talk at dinner, and she'd cry herself to sleep.

A typical teen might not have such intense mood swings, but you can be sure your teen will be moody. By definition, the teenage years are unstable. Bodies and minds are developing. Feelings of independence and dependence both want equal time. Friendships are rocky and constantly changing. And, if that wasn't enough, every September there's another school year—with new teachers, new classmates, and new expectations.

Margaret Mead coined the phrase "the generation gap" during the turbulent sixties. But clothing, behavior, and language are merely superficial trappings. As Dr. Daniel Offer and Dr. Michael Rutter have shown, teenagers and their parents enjoy a good relationship. In terms of politics, values, career expectations, and economic goals, they are very much alike—and neither views the other as a part of a widening "gap."

We adults see teenagers as our hope. If we view them as different from us, perhaps they can solve our society's problems and the world can be a better place.

But, in reality, teens might talk up a good storm, but they cannot change the world. They simply do not have enough knowledge or experience to make a difference.

Your teen might even blame his moods on you. For many teens, it's their parents who are erratic. Let's face it. One day you can be yelling at your son to clean up his room only to beam over his excellent report card the next. Think back on your teenage years, the way you felt when a teacher told you, "Good job!" or when you received your driver's license, the elation from that first kiss, or the pain from the fight with your best friend. Remember the intensity of your emotions—and how the feelings from these memories linger even today. Whether it's schoolwork, friendship, or a rite of passage, the situations teenagers face have the same impact as the stresses we adults feel. But teens do not have the experience or the maturity to cushion their blows. And their move through these peaks and valleys occurs almost on a daily basis.

The fact is that teens haven't learned to cope with life's ambivalence. They aren't quite sure what their strengths and their weaknesses are. They are still developing their sense of self. In time, teens will develop a clearer picture of life and they will become more even-tempered.

6. "I'm the Greatest!"

Janice loved to talk—about herself. She couldn't conceive of anything more riveting or entertaining. It wasn't simply conceit; it was the fact that she couldn't see any other point of view. She couldn't understand why her older brother was furious when she went into the bathroom before him every morning. She couldn't believe that her mother might want the car to do some errands—when all her high school friends were waiting for her at the mall.

Janice is a typical example of teenage egocentricity. As teens move further and further away from their parents, they need to restore that lost sense of self. Though friendships fill some of those empty self spaces, it's not enough. Their need to establish an identity is so great that they just don't have room for other people and for other problems—nor will they be able to see anything that doesn't correspond with their current view of the world.

Teenagers are bombarded by their developing minds and bodies from the inside and by new demands and responsibility from the outside. Focusing on his needs holds the teenager together and stops him from becoming overwhelmed. Keeping the "I" on center stage reduces his dependency on his parents, and it asserts his newfound separateness. His attitudes are different from his mom's and dad's. He is becoming his own person.

7. "If I Could Run the World . . ."

Sally was her own "great books" club. She loved to discuss the classics she was reading for English. She would carry on about the invasion of Normandy until the rest of her family almost fell asleep over their roast beef. She talked about her views of the world and its problems as if she alone had discovered them—and she alone could provide solutions.

Think of Sally's behavior as exercise for the brain. As we have seen in chapter one, adolescence brings a new, more sophisticated level of cognitive thinking. Teens can now understand abstract thoughts and the meaning behind proverbs and quotes. They can make analogies and come to conclusions using logic and deductive reasoning. And, in the same way that they will exercise their new muscles, teens will use their brain, testing their newfound skills over and over again until they've mastered them. They will also use their new cognitive skills to "show up" their parents, intellectually reinforcing their drive toward independence.

Not every teen has this burst of intellectual capability and, in those who do, it is short-lived. Time subdues its intensity. In fact, the greatest work of many of our composers and mathematicians has been done in late adolescence and early adulthood, while this intellectual capability is at its peak.

8. "Rebel with a Cause"

Remember Eileen, the girl I wrote about in the beginning of this chapter? She's the one who donned punk jewelry and spiked short hair—all the better to go with her black clothes and sullen stare. Eileen's parents couldn't figure out who this creature was who had invaded their house, but, in actuality, Eileen's "acting out" was acting normal. For some teens, rebellion translates into independence and freedom. It's a way to keep fear and confusion at bay. Acting out keeps teens busy—and prevents boredom. As Dr. Meeks says in *High Times/Low Times:* " 'I'm bored' is not simply a spoiled teen's lament. It is an anxious voice trying to stay one step ahead of fear."

On the other hand, there are teens who seem to avoid activity. Jason didn't look like a rebel. He'd quietly do his chores and his homework—before making a dash for his room. There, behind closed doors, he'd play his blues and his jazz—using earphones to shut out all other sounds.

But Jason too is a rebel—an introverted one. Pushing away the outside world is still acting out, but it is more passive. Both outward rebelliousness and introversion effectively keep the "inner enemy" of fear away. Both divert attention. Both Eileen's punk manner and Jason's isolation hide unacceptable emotions. If they act angry or sullen, they can disguise their "babyish" feeling of love and need for their parents.

9. "Wizards and Witches"

Give Dave a science fiction paperback and he'd devour it overnight. His favorite computer and video games were ones that take place in other worlds, where magic and sorcery help the hero on his quest. Though he'd never admit it to a soul, he even read his horoscope every day in the morning paper.

It's a fact: teenagers love fantasy. One only has to look at the success of movies like *Nightmare on Elm Street* or *Aliens* to know that, for teens (and for many a parent), a good horror flick is pure entertainment, not an embodiment of fear. Teens will go straight to the haunted house on the hill. They'll seek out fortune-tellers. They'll look for omens on the street. The supernatural holds demons that are black and white and easily identified. Fantasy and science fiction hold unknowns they can enjoy—and walk away from when they are done.

Above all, teenagers are individuals, human beings going through a spurt of emotional, physical, and mental growth that we, as parents, sometimes forget will make them vulnerable. Very soon, they will be expected to take their places in the adult world—without the wisdom of experience to help them handle their new roles. Ultimately, what's astonishing is not that some teens have problems, but that the majority don't. The fact is that *most teenagers go through adolescence unscathed and without any turmoil.*

A WORLD WITHOUT PAIN

Adolescent angst is almost a cliché. The recordings from writers in the past, the complaints from countless parents, the data from psychoanalysts over the years—all claim that adolescence is a difficult period.

And, in many ways, it's true. As we have seen, adolescents are grappling with their changing bodies, their forming selves, and their burgeoning sexuality. They are dealing with independence from their families, increased responsibility and abilities, career striving, and more. And many teens do go through a great deal of angst, displaying the behaviors I just finished describing in dramatic ways.

THE CLASSICS

"The most dangerous class of New Yorkers is its children!" So proclaimed reformer Charles Loring Brace in the late 1800s. He was prompted by the disorderly teenage gangs so prevalent on New York City streets—from the Dead Rabbits and the Bowery Boys to the Little Plug Uglies and the Forty Little Thieves.

Why so much disorderly conduct in what have been misconstrued as "the good old days"? Crowded and hot conditions at home. Child labor—with long, hard hours. Unbridled growth in industry—which didn't wait for society to catch up. "Overnight" wealth. A sense of adventure and promise.

Adapted from *High Times/Low Times: The Many Faces of Adolescent Depression,* which, in turn, was adapted from *Rites of Passage: Adolescents in America 1790 to the Present* by Joseph Kett, New York: Basic Books, 1977.

But generalizations can be dangerous. We parents are partially to blame. The passage of time tempers our perspective. It's difficult to remember our own teenage years. Furthermore, we can have unconscious or irrational feelings about our teens—from competitiveness and envy to eroticism—which cause conflicting emotions within us. We can also see in our kids "a second chance"—leading to our excessive criticism when we see "our" faults in them or to our bestowing unrealistic expectations on them that they can't possibly meet.

Society at large also has a lot to do with our view of teenagers. We have preconceived myths and notions of how teens should behave—and how they should grow. We tend to group all teens together, as if they were a strange minority subculture, instead of treating them as individual people. This attitude is perpetuated by the teens themselves. As we have seen earlier in this chapter, they do cluster in groups and hang out with each other.

Society itself has also changed. Teenagers today live in a vastly different world than even the one we grew up in a short twenty years or so ago. From corporate takeovers to the availability of dangerous and illegal drugs, from inflation to AIDS, from the immediacy of communication to the fierce competition for jobs, from sophisticated special effects to the violence on television and in films—all these help shape and condition our youth, and all require a way of coping that may be different from the way we handled things. For example, a teen who appears passive and "laid back" might be coping better with our fast-changing world than a teen who is steadfast in his views.

Finally, the specialists themselves help promote the idea of teenage angst. From Freud on, adolescence has been seen as a difficult time, fraught with anger and turmoil, a time when an internal war for selfhood rages within each boy and girl. But medical professionals only see adolescents with turmoil. In fact, studies show that in seven out of ten cases, mental health professionals describe normal adolescents as significantly more disturbed than the adolescents view themselves.

However, there is no doubt that a sense of self is paramount for healthy development. As we have seen, the striving for self is a crucial component of the adolescent years. In 1971 Dr. Heinz Kohut discovered that if a teen doesn't acknowledge the parts of his unconscious selves, it can lead to self-destructive behavior. Other psychiatrists postulated that low self-esteem occurred when there was a gap between a teen's idealized self and his perceived actual self, and that repressing feelings and attitudes from the self is the root of psychopathology. In fact, as Drs. Daniel Offer, Eric Ostrov, and Kenneth I. Howard wrote in their book *The Adolescent*: "An adolescent unable to acknowledge important self-feelings, unable to make accurate predictions about himself interpersonally, or unable to regard himself highly, could be seen as emotionally unhealthy."

But does a teen have to go through adolescent angst to create a healthy self-image? Does every adolescent grapple with the search for self like a warrior fighting a deadly beast? Can adolescents form an identity without turbulence and with relative comfort and ease? In short, is adolescent angst normal?

It was these questions that led Dr. Daniel Offer and his colleagues to embark on a long-term study of adolescents in 1960. Using the concept of self as the central issue of adolescence, Offer constructed a questionnaire that he brought to high schools across the country in the 1970s and 1980s.

Dr. Offer organized his Offer Self-Image Questionnaire (OSIQ) along five areas of self—because teens have feelings and attitudes about each one. The questionnaire itself was in a true or false format, with each teen marking the statements as he or she perceived them. The five areas were:

- *The Psychological Self.* This portion of the questionnaire included impulse control, emotional tone, and body and self-image, with statements such as: "I am proud of my body." "My feelings are easily hurt." "At times I have fits of crying and/or laughing that I seem unable to control."
- *The Social Self.* This part explored a teen's attitudes about social relationships, morals, and vocational and educational goals. Statements here included: "I like to help a friend whenever I can." "I enjoy most parties I go to." "I would rather be supported for the rest of my life than work."
- *The Sexual Self.* Here, sexual attitudes were analyzed in questions such as: "Dirty jokes are fun at times." "It is very hard for a teenager to know how to handle sex in a right way." "I often think about sex."
- *The Familial Self.* Adolescents in this portion considered questions about family relationships, including: "When I grow up and have a family, it will be in at least a few ways similar to my own." "My parents are usually patient with me." "Very often parents don't understand a person because they had an unhappy childhood."
- *The Coping Self.* The final portion of the questionnaire dealt with statements regarding mastery of the external world, possible psychopathology, and adjustment capabilities. Here's a sampling: "I

am confused most of the time." "When a tragedy occurs to one of my friends, I feel sad, too." "I do not have many fears which I cannot understand."

Here are the results of the groundbreaking six-year study:

The Psychological Self

On the whole, adolescents have a strong body image. Because they are physically healthy, they feel good about themselves. Fifty percent of the teens do experience anxiety, but this too is normal. This anxious state occurs only in new or unusual situations.

Most teens:

- Enjoy life
- Are happy with themselves most of the time
- Are healthy and strong
- Are self-confident
- Feel proud of their physical development

The Social Self

Girls, on the whole, were more concerned with the feelings of others than were boys. They were also more concerned with telling the truth. Boys felt like leaders more often than the girls and they were more autonomous.

Most teens:

- Believe they will feel proud of their future work
- Do not want to be supported forever
- Desire independence
- Believe there will be a job waiting for them when they are ready
- Enjoy the company of others
- Make friends easily

The Sexual Self

Most teens:

- Are not afraid of their sexuality or sexual feelings
- Find sex pleasurable

Incidentally, boys were found to be more open about their sexuality than girls.

The Familial Self
Most teens:

- Have a good relationship with family members
- Do not feel there is a "generation gap"
- Have no problems with their parents
- Are optimistic about future relationships

The Coping Self
Most teens:

- Can control themselves in most situations
- Are optimistic and hopeful about their future
- Are relaxed
- Have no feelings of inferiority
- Do not feel others treat them badly
- Are comfortable with their world and adjust well to it

THE SILENT MINORITY

Contrary to popular beliefs, teenagers are happier, more self-confident, and calmer than Fred MacMurray could ever have imagined for his three sons. As the OSIQ results prove, most adolescents go through their teenage years without turmoil.

But Dr. Offer and others have also found that, despite this optimistic report, 20 percent of all teenagers do suffer—and have inner turmoil. There are currently 18 million adolescents in the United States. Twenty percent translates into 3.6 million suffering teens. And 80 percent of these suffering teens suffer in silence.

I deal with troubled teens every day of my life. I see their worries, their pain, and their fear. I see the results of the suffering they had to deal with in silence for so long. If your child feels invisible, he or she needs your help. It is important to see past the clichés and your own preconceived notions and find the child silently crying out and struggling to adulthood.

We have now seen the normal side of adolescent life. It's time to switch sets and see if your child is in pain. It's time to recognize the signs and symptoms of trouble.

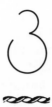

PAIN CUES:
Recognizing a Teen in Trouble

Parents are under a lot of pressure. Not only do they have to worry about providing food, shelter, and education—at a time when our economy is struggling—they must also serve as an early-warning system for the physical and mental health of their children. This task, especially understanding the emotional and psychological life of a troubled teen, is difficult for even a seasoned mental health professional. How, then, can parents recognize that their teens are in trouble? Well, it isn't easy, but a parent can, with enough insight—and luck—spot a troubled teen. I've devised the following quiz to help them.

IS YOUR TEEN STRUGGLING?

These statements are divided into the three potential trouble zones: home, school, and social activities. Each one describes a situation that can signal a problem. Look them over. Think about them. Mark each statement that you feel is true about your child—either through your own observation or through information you have received from a teacher, a doctor, a religious leader, or a neighbor. Some of the following statements seem quite harmless, and by themselves they usually don't indicate a problem. But taken together with other seemingly harmless statements they may provide an overall picture of a troubled teen. I must stress, however, that this quiz should never substitute for the professional diagnosis of a health-care provider. Please note that "your son" and "your daughter" are used interchangeably.

TROUBLE ZONE ONE: SCHOOL
1. My son's grades have been steadily slipping.
2. My daughter was just rejected from the college she wanted to attend.
3. My son's been cutting school.
4. My daughter is spending all her free time on her homework—instead of seeing her friends.
5. My son didn't make the football team.
6. My daughter's graduation is only a few weeks away.
7. My son has a high I.Q.—but you'd never know it from his grades.
8. My daughter complains about school inordinately.
9. My son's teacher called me in to talk about his disorderly conduct in class.
10. My daughter's been crying herself to sleep for the past week because she didn't get an "A" on a recent paper.
11. My son wants to drop out of school.
12. My daughter refuses to do her homework.
13. My son has a consistent "A" average, but he's still terrified he'll fail.
14. My daughter refuses to wake up in the morning. I literally have to push her out the door to get her to school on time.
15. My son said he was too sick to go to school this morning—for the eighth time this month.

TROUBLE ZONE TWO: HOME
1. My spouse and I both work hard—and there never seems to be enough time for the family to be together.
2. My son stays in his room night after night with the door closed tight.
3. My daughter is never home.
4. No one ever calls my son on the phone.
5. My daughter always has a lot of friends over to the house—but they're never the same ones.

6. My son likes to hang around with our friends—instead of kids his own age.
7. My spouse died a year ago.
8. My daughter refuses to listen to me.
9. My son won't talk to me.
10. My daughter never cleans her room.
11. My son doesn't seem to sleep. His light stays on the whole night long.
12. My daughter doesn't like to shower and her hair is always limp and dirty.
13. My son has been waking up from terrible nightmares.
14. My daughter isn't as popular as her older sister.
15. My son is preoccupied with the idea of death.
16. My daughter keeps saying, "I don't care"—about everything.
17. My son's gotten very moody. He gets down at the drop of a hat.
18. My daughter has recently lost too much weight.
19. My son looks up to his older brother—and wants to do and be exactly like him.
20. My spouse and I have just separated—and the kids seem to be in shock.
21. Every night, my daughter plays the same sad song over and over and over again.
22. My son throws temper tantrums for no reason. Yesterday, he almost broke a window.
23. My daughter has taken to screaming—at everyone in the family.
24. My divorce is finally official.
25. A close relative has just died.
26. My son puts his headphones on every night and listens to music for hours at a time.
27. My daughter mopes around the house. She doesn't seem interested in anything.
28. My son keeps making jokes about suicide.

TROUBLE ZONE THREE: SOCIAL ACTIVITIES

1. My daughter keeps to a rigid—and exhaustive—exercise routine.
2. My son has gotten three speeding tickets in the last month.
3. My spouse has a drinking problem.
4. My daughter is amazing: she is on five school committees, three community service organizations—and she's the president of her graduating class. All this and a straight "A" student, too. Even

though she seems to be doing fine, I'm a little worried. I don't know how she handles everything.

5. We just moved to a new town—and the kids don't like it.
6. My son broke his leg last winter—and he's been in a cast ever since.
7. My daughter is starting to dress much too provocatively.
8. My son just lost his best friend in a car accident.
9. My daughter might be pregnant.
10. My son stopped seeing his friends.
11. My daughter has been home from school all fall with a bout of mono—and she's just about ready to go back.
12. A classmate committed suicide.
13. My spouse can get abusive.
14. My daughter's boyfriend just broke up with her.
15. My son has dropped all the things he used to love to do.
16. My daughter lives on cottage cheese and diet soda—but I've seen her gobble a bag of chocolate chip cookies in one fell swoop.
17. My son just wrecked the family car.
18. My daughter has a glazed look in her eyes and she acts like she's on another planet.
19. I found a bottle of pills in my son's room.
20. My daughter's smoking cigarettes on the sly.
21. My son has a group of new friends—and none of them go to his school.
22. My daughter breaks out in a rash whenever she gets invited to a party.
23. My son never goes out on dates. He says he hasn't met anyone he likes.
24. My daughter wears the same jeans and sweatshirt day after day—and she has no desire to go shopping for other clothes.

These statements are only generalizations. But if you've checked several of them, it is possible that your teenager is suffering—and having problems that go beyond the normal slings and arrows of adolescent life. I urge you to speak to your child—and to your physician—if any number of them ring true.

As with any emotion, pain is complicated; there are as many levels and reasons as there are ways to react. Your teenager's suffering can be the result of both genetic and environmental influences—which surface as one or several different types of disorders. On the other hand, your teen's suffering can be a normal and healthy reaction to pain—and not be a cause for alarm.

To understand your child's pain, you must understand its source.

WHEN SUFFERING IS NORMAL

"What do I want to make of myself and what do I have to work with?" Erik Erikson found this to be the compelling question of the teenage years. We have seen how most teens face this question with enthusiasm and confidence. But even the most healthy teen will occasionally feel some anxiety, depression, and irrationality because:

The push and pull of independence versus dependence can leave teens with a nagging, empty feeling. They want freedom, but they're losing the nourishing self-esteem they had always received from their parents.

The importance and fragility of teenage friendships is fertile ground for rejection. The self-oriented, insecure nature of peer issues almost guarantees that, sooner or later, a teen will get hurt.

Fluctuating mood swings can set a trap for despair. As we have seen in chapter one, ambivalence is a teenager's nightmare. Learning to live with shades of gray takes maturity and time. Instead, teens will fly high when they achieve success, spiral down when they fail—and get caught on a pendulum of anxiety between the two.

The vast physical, emotional, and mental changes teens experience can assault their self-esteem. Change can be exciting, exhilarating—and terrifying. Unpredictable body development, heightened sexual impulses, untested independence, added responsibility, uncharted territory—all chip away at the stability teenagers had as children, at the nourishment they had as satellites in their parent's universe. These vast sea changes are also felt more acutely in girls than boys. Studies have shown that girls in early adolescence are particularly susceptible to anxiety and depression. The onset of menstruation, bringing with it new, monthly hormonal changes, dramatically affects their moods. Socially and emotionally, many girls are still unconsciously taught to be "good" and to help others. The normal adolescent feelings of independence and selfishness are in direct contradiction—and can make them feel more guilty and resentful.

The instability and vulnerability of the teenage years adds fuel to suffering's flames. Growing up is very complicated—especially today, when adolescence can continue throughout a person's twenties. Years ago, adolescence began at puberty (around twelve for girls and around fourteen for boys) and ended with financial independence—which more times than not meant at eighteen or nineteen years of age. But many youths now go on to college and graduate school—and many of them need financial support from their parents well into their twenties. Further, many teens wait to marry and become parents themselves. Though physically mature, these young adults can still be going through a vast ocean of emotion and mental change. Inside, they can still be in the process of "growing up"—with its inherent struggle for independence and dependence, its mood swings, its fragile friendships, and its instability. Unfortunately, the outward maturity many young adults show the world hides an inner confusion—which continues to mount in silence as more and more adult responsibility is heaped on them.

Adolescents will get depressed—just as we do. A move to a new, strange neighborhood. The death of a loved one. A separation or divorce. Rejection—in any guise. All will cause pain. All will make your teen depressed.

It is natural to suffer after a loss or a change. Think of the last time you faced a painful situation. Let's say your project was turned down at work. Maybe you acted out, kicking your wastebasket in the privacy of your office. Maybe you broke down in tears. Maybe you went out drinking. But whether your behavior was childlike or mature, eventually you settled down. Your pain diminished. And the support and attention you received from your colleagues and your friends went a long way to easing your frustration.

The same holds true for our teens. The situation might be different, but the feelings are just as real. If your teen is upset about not making the honor roll, it's possible she will regress—kicking her bed or banging a locker door. She might cry in her pillow. She might demand more of your time, whining to get your attention and staying underfoot. But, eventually, in a few weeks' time, life will get better. Your teen will accept the loss. Slowly, your teen will go back out in the world, full of that adolescent hope and enthusiasm.

But sometimes the pain has a life of its own. Sometimes a teen does not bounce back. Instead of healing over time, the suffering gets worse.

. . . AND WHEN IT ISN'T

A crisis can bring out the best in people—or the worst. Disorders that have been lying dormant can surface. A response to an external situation can turn inward, becoming a two-headed monster of hate—at oneself and at the world at large.

The key thing to look for is change: in behavior, in attitude, and in physical appearance and function. Here are the seven general symptoms that signal trouble.

Changes in Behavior

1. LOSS OF INTEREST. You used to rant and rave about the way your son played his video games, morning, noon, and night. But lately they've just been gathering dust. Your daughter, on the other hand, stopped calling her friends a few weeks ago. Instead of chattering on the phone for hours, she's staring at the TV. From school to shopping malls, hobbies to hanging out with friends, a loss of interest in activities your teenager used to love is a common symptom of suffering.

Parent's pain cue: Look for any change in your teen's activity patterns that don't make sense to you.

2. CHANGES IN SCHOOL PERFORMANCE. Once upon a time, your son was a model student. But his grades have begun to slip and he doesn't seem to care. Or maybe your daughter is studying as much as she always has, but she just can't seem to concentrate. And her grades don't reflect the time she puts into her homework. Whether a drop in grades, an inability to concentrate, or simply a shift in attitude about school, changes in school performance signal trouble up ahead.

Parent's pain cue: Look for slipping grades, truancy, and homework that never seems to get done.

Changes in Attitude

3. DRAMATIC CHANGES IN MOOD. Every parent has seen it: When something good happens, he's on top of the world. When something bad happens, the world suddenly topples and crumbles at his feet. Mood swings are a part of a teenager's development. They stem from the uncertainty faced by a teenager as he begins to find self-worth through his own actions, not through the acceptance of his parents. But very dramatic changes of mood are *not* normal—especially when they last for a period of weeks. A teenager who becomes angry and irritable, stomping around the house and slamming doors, is not acting in a normal and healthy way. Neither is a teen who becomes sullen and quiet—only to snap at you if you ask what's wrong.

Parent's pain cue: Look out for any cranky, irritable, sad, or irrational display of emotion in your teen.

4. SUICIDAL THOUGHTS. It's a cruel, hard fact: A troubled teen will think about death. From self-injury strategies to self-inflicted punishments, adolescents in pain—like their adult counterparts—can become preoccupied with suicide. These suicidal thoughts go hand in hand with depression and excessive guilt feelings. A depressed teenager might think he made a fool of himself in front of others and take it to heart. He might take responsibility for bad things that happen to others. He might imagine a situation much worse than it is, become obsessive about it, or even create it out of thin air.

Parent's pain cue: Any reference to death, no matter how obscure, must be taken seriously. Unfortunately, it is not always easy to see the signs of suicidal thoughts. Teenagers rarely ask for help directly. Look for any change in attitude, especially if it is combined with sadness, obsessive chatter, self-denigration, and withdrawal.

Troubled boys will not talk about suicide; they'll only ask for help indirectly—by acting out or retreating. Asking for help is a sign of weakness to them, especially if they hang around a great deal with other boys. In fact, they won't try to commit suicide as often as girls, but boys are three times more likely to succeed if they do try.

Troubled girls, however, are more open. They will talk about their feelings with you and their friends. But even conversation doesn't always work and the stress from their pain can continue to build. Girls will attempt suicide three times more often than boys. However, they are less likely to die from their actions.

Changes in Physical Appearance and Body Functions

5. SLEEP DISTURBANCES. We all know the results of insomnia. Tossing and turning the whole night through is a common symptom of trouble for adults. But troubled teenagers, on the whole, suffer from hypersomnia. They will sleep much *more* than they usually do—and, when they finally do wake up, they'll feel tired, foggy, and unfocused. However, as the day progresses, they'll begin to feel better—and stay up late. Unfortunately, parents usually blame this new sleep pattern on late-night habits—and not on the pain. The teenagers too are at fault. They will point to their schoolwork, their parents, or their "excessive" responsibility as the cause of their tiredness—instead of examining the very real suffering they feel inside.

Parent's pain cue: Look for any sign of unexplained fatigue—from an inability to get up in the morning to low energy, from constant complaints to edginess.

6. WEIGHT CHANGE. Some teens will just stop eating. Others will gobble up everything in sight and immediately throw it all up. Still others will eat morning, noon, and night without coming up for air. Excessive weight loss or weight gain are both signs of trouble, especially when combined with compulsive eating habits.

Parent's pain cue: Look for any weight change in your teen—as well as different eating habits and attitudes about food.

7. MOVEMENT AND COORDINATION DISTURBANCES. Your son might start the day heavy and lethargic—only to be poetry in motion by nightfall. Your daughter might start and end her days in slow motion, but the afternoon will find her agitated and fidgety. On the other hand, your teenager might be a study in uncoordination, breaking dishes, stepping over feet, or knocking into furniture. When a teenager's emotions are erratic, swinging back and forth from feelings of grandeur and failure, they will be reflected in his movements and in his muscular coordination.

Parent's pain cue: Look for erratic, changeable movement or clumsy coordination.

Unfortunately, understanding these seven signs of trouble is not enough. Teenagers are masters of disguise, camouflaging their pain from you—and themselves. In order for you to recognize the symptoms of pain in your teen, you must also see beyond the disguises to the real performance underneath. Here are five different masks troubled teens may wear, and one that parents often wear.

Number One: The Mask of Ordinary Life
There is a fine line between a teen in pain and a teen suffering the normal disturbances of adolescent life. How can you recognize the difference? As Dr. Meeks notes, "Take note of the duration and severity of your child's symptoms. Trust your instincts. Try to communicate. And don't hesitate to seek professional advice."

Number Two: The Mislabeled Mask
Even adults can have difficulty pinpointing a problem. Without adult knowledge or experience, teens have an even harder time identifying the source of their pain. Instead of recognizing their inner struggle, they

will blame the outside world. Instead of saying, "I feel sad," a troubled teen might say, "I'm bored." And, if you were to ask your troubled child point-blank if she is having a problem, her answer might sound like this: "Yeah, I'm having some problems, but it's only because school is a complete drag. I hate it." Teens are focused on action, not words. They are programmed to impatiently plunge in and *do,* not to question themselves. They cannot see that it's their inner pain that makes their school, family, or friends so distasteful.

Number Three: The Mask of Independence
"Mom, I'm scared. I need your help." If only a parent of a troubled teen could hear those words! Unfortunately, direct cries for help are rare. Teens are trying to break away from their parents and, to their minds, asking for help means needing them too much. Reaching out for help is "for babies," a move backward to that childish dependency they are instinctively trying to escape. Further, troubled teens can't always recognize the need for help in themselves. Instead, they'll put on false bravado, pretending they can handle anything that comes along. But inside, their troubled souls are silently crying.

Number Four: The Mask of Achievement
As we have seen, it isn't easy for teens to recognize the fact that they are having problems. They only know they are hurting—but they aren't sure why. Unfortunately, many teens conclude that they are feeling bad because they *are* bad. Instead of saying, "I have a problem," they'll say, "I'm worthless. I'm nothing." In order to alleviate these negative feelings, some teens will do more and more, trying to be perfect in every aspect of their lives. By overachieving, they can do better than anyone else. By doing better than anyone else, they can feel worthy. On the other hand, some teens turn their negative feelings into a self-fulfilling prophecy. They are nothing—so they will do nothing. By underachieving, they reaffirm their belief that they are worthless. But neither overachieving nor underachieving gets to the source of the problem. Peel away this mask and you will find a very troubled, scared teen.

Number Five: The Mask of Excitement
Anxiety and pain need an outlet. If a teen denies his pain, it must go somewhere. And nothing fits the bill better for the active and impressionable teen than excitement. Fear provides the fuel to keep "one step ahead" of troubling thoughts. Unfortunately, this need for excitement leads many teens down a dangerous path of self-destructive behavior.

It is a time when they might begin experimenting with drugs to cover up their painful symptoms—and I'll be discussing this later.

Number Six: The Mask That Parents Wear
Denial is a potent tool. No parent likes to see his or her child in pain. A father who was a football star in high school won't want to see that his son absolutely hates the sport. A mother who was once "the belle of the ball" will have trouble seeing that no one is asking her daughter out. The same holds true for psychological problems. Parents will unconsciously ignore the signs. Further, if they are having problems themselves, they won't be able to see past their own pain—or their own unresolved adolescent issues. Other members of the family will deny the simmering trouble as well. Families are resistant to change; there is an instinctual "pecking order" and change—in any guise—can threaten the balance and the continuation of the family group. Even normal teens will feel their family's tug as they gradually move from dependence to independence. For troubled teens, that tug is increased tenfold. They can't express their feelings for fear of destroying the status quo. Ditto the other family members. Instead of acknowledging the troubled teen, they will deny him, sweeping his problems under the rug. Depression, substance abuse, eating disorders—all are too painful, too strange for many families to face. "We'll manage," they'll say and smile, putting up a good front—as the pain the troubled teen is feeling begins to permeate the entire family structure, as the trouble begins to infect everyone.

These are the symptoms and the disguises teens in trouble will display. It is now time to turn to why—why suffering can become abnormal and why some teens develop psychological problems.

THE TROUBLED FACE BEHIND THE MASK

Some would call it genetic predisposition. Some would call it a product of environment and childhood development. Others would point to temperament and the ability to cope with life's ups and downs. And still others would call it the luck of the draw. In actuality, the reasons why some teenagers develop psychological problems are a combination of all of these factors.

Some teens might already have a genetic predisposition to a psychiatric illness: a depressed mother, a grandparent suffering from anxiety, a manic-depressive father. Studies of adopted twins show that even though their children were reared by different families, genetic predispositions surfaced.

But predisposed to does not mean predetermined. The environment also plays a part in whether or not a predisposition becomes a reality. One particular study of fifty abused children found that 40 percent of them had emotional disturbances. But once they were removed from their abusive environment, these children made physical and intellectual progress.

Childhood development also has a role in adolescent performance. Proper physiological and neurological growth. Solid emotional attachments. Cognitive stimulation and support. Encouragement and permission to explore the world outside the cradle. Consistent moral and social training. An easy temperament. Like a building with a strong foundation, these positive childhood factors can help make the replay of development during adolescence a smash hit—or a flop. They can provide the tools for a teenager to overcome a crisis—or be swallowed up by its pain.

Here's an example: A study discussed by Dr. Marian Radke-Yarrow in an article by Daniel Goleman in *The New York Times* found that children with depressed parents became depressed not because of genetic factors, but because of the way the depressed mother or father interacted with them. The study found that:

- Depressed mothers are more likely to back off when they meet resistance from children while trying to control them.
- Depressed mothers are less able to compromise in disagreements with their children, and they often confused their children's normal attempts at independence as rule-breaking.
- While making and eating lunch, the depressed mothers spoke to their children far less than did other mothers.
- When the depressed mothers did speak to their children, they made more negative comments.

Researchers have long tried to determine whether genetics, childhood development, or environment is the most important—to no avail. The basic truth that has come out of all this controversy is this: If one or both parents have a disorder, their child will be at a greater risk of developing it himself. However, this predisposition will surface only if the child's development and environment provide the soil.

But I have also added another component: stress. If a child's coping capabilities have been developed in strong and healthy ways, the environment will not affect her—predisposition or not. But if that same child has difficulty coping with life's problems, a disorder can take seed—even if there is no history of that disorder in her family. Children from impoverished or broken homes can come out relatively unscarred. Disadvantaged children can come out healthier than children of wealthier, loving parents.

It all comes down to stress—and how well a child handles it. The fact is that genetic predispositions can become reality only with stress. Environmental issues can influence a problem's appearance only if there is stress. Childhood development can lead the way to a disorder only if it has been paved with stress. Depression, anxiety, conduct disorder, anorexia, and other adolescent problems all have their roots in stress.

STRESS: THE NUMBER-ONE PAIN CUE

A fact: If you are alive, you will feel stress at some time or another in your life. And, contrary to popular belief, it is not the stress that is harmful. It is how you cope with stress that makes it bad. As Dr. Andrew Slaby said in his book *Aftershock: Surviving the Delayed Effects of Trauma, Crisis and Loss,* "Stress can be the thing that pushes us over the edge or the springboard to growth and opportunity."

For adults, stress can come from negative situations like getting fired, experiencing the death of a loved one, and divorce. It can also come from positive things: promotions, marriage, and birth.

Teenagers experience the same sense of stress as adults—and, as with adults, resiliency, strength, and good support systems can help them weather their storms. But, unlike adults, they lack the wisdom, perception, and experience of maturity to help them cope. Adults will usually be able to recognize the signs of stress and verbalize them. Teenagers, as we have seen, have a different point of view of the world. They will not verbalize their feelings in the same way—and they might not recognize stress for what it is. An adult might say: "This job is killing me. I'm completely stressed out. I think it's time to look around." But a teen might internalize the effects of stress, thinking: "School is driving me crazy. I don't know what to do. Everyone else is getting 'A's. It must be my fault. It's all my fault."

Teens are also affected by different stresses than adults. Before we go on, take a moment to do this quiz. It lists various situations that cause stress in teenagers. See if any of them pertain to your child.

YOUR TEEN MIGHT BE UNDER STRESS IF . . .
 1. He has been laid up with a football injury.
 2. She broke up with her steady boyfriend.

3. He failed a midterm test.
4. She doesn't understand geometry.
5. He has trouble understanding what he's reading.
6. You are in the process of a divorce.
7. You are remarrying—or your ex is.
8. Someone close has just died.
9. You are feeling tired and out of sorts.
10. The family has just moved to a new neighborhood.
11. Graduation is just around the corner.
12. She is leaving the familiar corridors of junior high for the county high school.
13. He is recuperating from mono.
14. She is pregnant.
15. He just had a fight with his best friend.
16. You and your spouse have been fighting.
17. Your spouse has recently lost a job.
18. Your new baby has just been brought home.
19. She has to give a speech in front of the entire student body.
20. Summer vacation is here.
21. He just got accepted into college.
22. She's the only one of her friends who made cheerleading.
23. He was just turned down for a date.
24. She isn't going to the prom.
25. He was just voted "Most Likely to Succeed."

Dr. E. S. Kessler once said, "It is difficult to conceive of a human being progressing from infancy through adolescence without trauma sufficient to interfere, at least temporarily, with psychosocial development." The statements above reflect only a few of the "sufficient traumas" that can cause adolescent stress, but they can give you an idea of both the positive and negative circumstances that provide the fuel for adolescent stress—and its subsequent pain.

Basically, all adolescent stress stems from four different sources. Stress from all four sources can combine to trigger psychological problems. Let's go over each one now:

Biology
"The kids at school didn't like me because I was small. They beat me up and laughed at me. I didn't have any friends until I came to Fair Oaks Hospital." That's fifteen-year-old Dennis talking in one of our Performance Groups. He is currently at Fair Oaks for having tried to

commit suicide three times. He is suffering from depression, violent behavior, and a visual learning disability. The roots of his problems are deeper than simply physical appearance, but his small physique and abnormal biological development are a contributing factor. They are a catalyst for the stress he has already experienced in life—and a trigger for his pain.

It makes sense. Studies have shown that physical development can affect other areas of development. A boy who is physically immature won't be asked to participate in sports—and he'll have a harder time getting dates. A girl who physically matures too quickly will be asked out more often by boys—without the emotional development to handle sex. She might not be as trusted or well-liked by other girls. Additional studies have shown that when girls and boys physically mature early, parents and teachers will expect them to do more—even if they aren't equipped to handle it cognitively or emotionally.

The ultimate result of early or late maturation is stress. And without good coping skills and a good support system, this stress can trigger depression, loneliness, and self-destructive behavior.

Another factor is a teenager's looks. As we have seen in chapter two, early adolescence is fraught with superficial friendships. So much of a teenager's self-esteem comes from his peers—who, in turn, will accept him because of his physical appearance. An overweight girl will have few dates. A small boy, like Dennis above, will be tormented by his peers. A plain-looking girl will not be popular—regardless of her grade-point average. A study of five hundred juvenile delinquents and five hundred nondeliquents by Drs. Glueck and Glueck found that 60 percent of the juvenile delinquents had heavier and thicker muscles and bones. Another study found that delinquent girls were shorter, fatter, and more muscular than female college students.

Eventually, in most cases, things even out and superficiality is dropped for more valuable assets. But physical appearance can add stress—and lead to possible scars in later life.

Biology also becomes a stressor when learning disabilities and slight brain abnormalities are present. But environment can offset heredity. A study of minimally brain-damaged infants found that 18 percent of these children who came from unstable families grew up to have long-term psychiatric problems. But only 2 to 3 percent of the children from stable homes grew up with problems. Further, studies have not been able to prove that brain abnormalities such as epilepsy have any impact on a child's later psychological development.

But physical illness or handicap, constitutional fragility, and brain impairment can cause their own brand of stress. Drug side effects, hospital admission, physical activity restriction, special treatment from family and peers—all have their effects on a growing child.

Teens suffering from brain abnormalities and learning disabilities can also be frustrated in school. Unfortunately, the stress from this frustration can lead not only to poorer grades and lower self-esteem, but also to possible aggressive behavior—and I will be discussing learning disabilities in greater detail in chapter six.

Family

"I look back and think about how horrible my past was and wish that it had never happened. It is very hard for me to accept the fact that I'm not living with the people I really love and care about—my birth parents." This is Jean, a fourteen-year-old girl in the Performance Group who had been shunted from family to family—and who was sexually and physically abused by one of her adoptive parents.

It is an understatement to say that Jean's family life has been stressful. Nor is it surprising to learn that she has tried to kill herself several times.

We have already seen how parents play a pivotal role in childhood—creating a climate in which emotional, cognitive, and social growth is either encouraged or allowed to flounder. But their influence doesn't stop at twelve. Families are crucial to a teenager's normal development. And, as many of us can attest, their presence can be felt throughout our lives. Because of their importance, it makes sense that families are a prime stage setting for stress. Jean's case might be an extreme example, but every family has its stress-making potential.

Families are dynamic. Roles, attitudes, and actions change with time, with life's rites and passages, with events in the outside world. In their book, *The Changing Family Life Cycle: A Framework for Family Therapy,* Betty Carter and Monica McGoldrick state that "family stress is often greatest at transition points from one stage to another of the family development process." These stages include:

- Marriage
- Birth
- Raising children
- The departure of children from the home
- Retirement
- Death

All of these stages signal change—which, in turn, brings stress. A new baby brings new responsibility—and changes the relationships between family members. A child approaching adolescence becomes more independent, creating new rules and establishing different boundaries. A teenager going off to college leaves an empty space.

Child care has become the parental stress of the nineties. The process of separation and individuation is made even more difficult when both mother and father go off to work each day. And their numbers are growing every day:

Sixty-five percent of American mothers have jobs that take them outside the home—and 55 percent have children under age six. Over 3 million children have mothers who return to work before the child is a year old. By 1990, only 14 percent of American households had just one working spouse.

"Warehouse parenting" is what Dr. Nina R. Lief calls the result of the question: "Who's bringing up baby when mom and dad are at work?" She feels that today's day-care centers do not offer acceptable care. She also believes that children under three cannot tolerate separation from their mothers—and an absence of six hours or more can psychologically harm an infant.

But other studies show that children are not necessarily traumatized when both mother and father go off to work. Despite the fact that their weekday routines are shared with a responsible nanny, au pair, or housekeeper, kids always recognize their parents—providing their parents spend time with them in the morning and at night. This is especially true if child care takes place in the child's home environment.

Here are some recommendations for better-quality child care from Dr. Lief:

- Expand training programs for caretakers
- Upgrade caretaker salaries
- Establish parenting groups
- Recognize parenting as a career—with financial compensation for mothers who elect to stay home
- Involve mental health professionals in the day-care issue

But there are other stress-makers in the home. One is in the relationships between family members. Parents influence their children and children will influence their parents—and relationships between family members will influence everyone. The way a husband and wife act with each other will affect the way they act with their children. The way a brother and sister act with each other will affect their parent's interaction. Tension and friction between family members can cause stress— and it can pass from one relationship to another.

Marital problems pay a heavy family stress toll. Divorce is as volatile for children as it is for adults. It changes and disrupts the family order. Everything is new and vulnerable. Attitudes, rules, and behavior change for everyone. But contrary to popular belief, divorce itself is not as harmful to children as the parental conflict and tension that comes with it. According to a study done by Dr. Michael Rutter in 1971, the disturbed relationships between family members signaled more problems than the actual process of separation. In fact, family discord was found to cause more delinquency and conduct disorder than the death of a parent. Unfortunately, divorce can increase family discord beyond the actual signing of the papers. Custody battles, changing financial status, family adjustment—all create a ripe atmosphere for stress and subsequent emotional problems. Studies bear this out: Behavior has been shown to worsen in the year after a marriage breaks up. But there is a happy ending: Research has proven that the effects of divorce are not irreversible. When home life once again quiets down and everyone has readjusted, problems subside. Within two years, adolescents with emotional and behavioral problems have shown improvement.

Discord, more than divorce, is the enemy. If parents are depressed or always at odds, their supervision can become haphazard. They might become more self-centered, offering less praise for good behavior and more dramatic responses to bad behavior. They will give conflicting messages to their children—and convey negative feelings much more often. They won't communicate with their children as easily. And, most importantly, they might fight over the children themselves: yelling at each other on child-raising matters, using the children as pawns in their battles, or taking out their hostility for each other on the kids.

A family's size also plays a role in stress. The larger the family, the less communication between parent and child. It isn't possible to give each child the attention or discipline he needs. Larger families are usually associated with poverty and overcrowding. Studies have found that teenagers who come from families with four or more children have less verbal intelligence and are at greater risk for developing conduct disorders (see chapter seven for more information). Only children have been found to have better verbal skills—possibly because they are given all their parents' attention.

Other stress-making family matters include: socioeconomic class, the physical health of each member, the extended family, ethnical and cultural backgrounds, and parental attitudes and beliefs.

School

"I hate school. The teachers didn't like me, the other kids didn't want to be my friends, and I was always getting punished for something that wasn't my fault." Ray is fifteen and, as a member of the Performance Group, he's gone back to the environment that once gave him so much pain.

Think of school as an office. For a teenager, the hallowed halls are as stressful as an adult's day on the job. It is a place where teens must prove themselves in class—and among their peers. They must meet homework deadlines. They are a part of a "team"—either in sports, in extracurricular activities, or in academic competitions. And all this on an almost daily basis!

Further, studies show that many teenagers have trouble adjusting to the transition from small, neighborhood elementary schools to large junior highs where teachers, students, and classes change all day long. As Lawrence Kutner wrote in his *New York Times* "Parent & Child" column, "The combination of new hormones and new homerooms can lead to emotional upset."

There are eight factors of school life that can go far in reducing adolescent stress:

1. A good balance between more- and less-intelligent students.
2. Generous use of rewards, praise, and appreciative support.
3. A comfortable, secure school atmosphere.
4. Ample opportunities for the students to share in the responsibilities and organization of the school.
5. A supportive and clear emphasis on academic performance.
6. Teachers who are encouraging, enthusiastic, and available to talk to students.
7. Organized, clear classroom rules and routines.
8. A staff that works together, agreeing on policies and curriculum.

Social Activities

"One reason I feel like I don't have any friends is because I push people away by being dramatic and annoying. The reason I act this way is because when I'm around people I get nervous and I have a lot of anxiety." Sixteen-year-old Joanne is not alone. When she talked about herself at one of our Performance Groups, many of the teenagers in the audience nodded their heads. They listened and understood.

The term "social activity" conjures up stress for many adolescents—and many adults as well. New people, new surroundings, new conversations . . . all have their place in the stress-making machinery of the social world.

This stage setting is really an offshoot of the three above. A family gathering can be a place of anxiety for an adolescent living in discord. An after-school meeting or dance can fill with dread the teen terrified of rejection. A physical handicap or chronic illness can make a biologically stressed-out teen self-conscious and unhappy in any social setting.

The best defense against stress in social situations is self-confidence and a good self-image. An article by Charles B. Irwin and Elaine Vaughan in the *Journal of Adolescent Health Care* makes the following recommendations for healthy psychosocial adolescent development:

- A supportive family environment that allows independence in small, graded steps.
- An atmosphere at home, at school, and among peers that rewards and supports positive risk-taking, encourages trying out new ideas, and accepts mistakes.
- An ongoing mutuality and respect between teens and significant adults.

There is power in numbers—and the whole can be greater than its parts. One has only to look at cults, clubs, or a book such as *Lord of the Flies,* where group consciousness proved stronger than civilized individuality, to see its potency. Another example: A study called "Robber's Cave" by Dr. Muzafer Sherif and his colleagues brought a group of eleven-year-old boys together for an experimental summer camp. None of the boys knew each other when they first came to the camp, but, within a few days, they'd all broken down into small tight groups. The ties within each clique became so strong so quickly that intense competition and tension between the groups emerged. It was only when the boys were asked to do something as a whole for the camp at large that cooperation and peace were seen. The moral? Social forces have a life of their own and it is the nature of a particular social activity that creates negative or positive stress—and subsequent negative or positive behavior.

These are the stage settings where stress plays—sometimes daily, sometimes only occasionally, and sometimes for a continuous long run.

As we have seen, it is not the stress itself but the way teens handle it that makes them strong and more self-confident—or triggers within them a psychological disorder.

Studies have shown that extremely stressful traumas—such as a move, a hospital stay, or the birth of a sibling—in the first four years of life predispose an adolescent to psychological problems when stressful situations occur in the teenage years.

But even if a teen does not experience trauma in those early years, a major life stress during adolescence can still precipitate problems. Studies have shown that the loss of a loved one, the threat of loss (such as a life-threatening illness or possible divorce), or a perceived failure (such as failing in an important test or being rejected by a close friend) have all been recently experienced by many depressed and suicidal teens—regardless of their early life stresses.

On the other hand, I have seen many teenagers who have lived through intense stress come out relatively unscathed. The fact is that some teenagers are better equipped to handle stress. Their coping capabilities are intact and they can better adjust to new circumstances. Daniel Goleman, in *The New York Times,* recently discussed the case of a six-year-old diabetic girl whose mother was severely depressed and whose father was an alcoholic. Though this young girl lived with ongoing stress, she was, by age nine, cheerful, well-liked, and an excellent student to boot. Why? Like other children who have grown up healthy despite stressful experiences, she had:

- *A good support system.* Neighbors and other children can supply the social and emotional needs not met by parents.
- *A good temperament.* A warm, smiling and easy child will make friends easily. She can become the "shining star" in a parent's otherwise depressing life—and grow up feeling special and needed.
- *Resiliency.* The strength and ability to act and to adjust to changing circumstances goes far in reducing stress.

Coping skills are inherent in each individual. But they can also be taught—which is one of the roles of therapy.

Stress in adolescents is particularly challenging because at the same time teens are suffering from a stressful situation, they are still developing. Their minds and bodies are growing, but their perceptions and their reactions to stress are stuck in the past. This creates additional stress and confusion, which, more times than not, causes teens to "act out" in destructive ways.

Here's an example. Sally's stepfather physically abused her when she was only five years old. At that age, she could only see herself as "bad," a girl who needed to be punished. She thought she was in the wrong— not her stepfather. Now she's fourteen and trying to cope with the stresses of adolescent life. But inside she still feels like that "bad" little girl; her self-esteem is nil. When her boyfriend broke up with her, it was because she was obnoxious. When she didn't pass a test, it was because she didn't deserve to get a passing grade. These negative responses to stress after stress began to weigh her down. The only way she felt she could cope was with suicide, and she attempted it three times before she came to Fair Oaks Hospital.

In order for troubled teens to become healthy, both the actual disorders and the underlying stress must be treated—and I'll be going over the therapeutic processes in subsequent chapters.

In short, stress can be harmful. But it's important to remember that some stress is good—and necessary for growth. Without the stress that comes with new, unknown situations, there would be no challenge and no risk. No child would strive to become independent or seek out new ideas. No child would dare to dream.

COMMON DISORDERS FOUND IN ADOLESCENTS

I've often been asked what I believe is the most common problem teenagers face today—and I always give the same answer: growing up and accepting themselves for who they are.

This problem, in turn, can give rise to self-doubt, fear, low self-esteem, and insecurity. What emerges from this fear and confusion are the various adolescent disorders: depression, eating disorders, substance abuse, anxiety disorders, and more.

Teens usually suffer from more than one disorder. Many of them overlap—and camouflage other disorders. Drug abuse can mask depression, anxiety, or other psychiatric disorders. A learning disability can result in depression—and require a different treatment. An eating disorder can go hand in hand with depression, drug abuse, and anxiety disorders. If you feel your teen is having problems, it's crucial you seek professional advice. Only a physician can give you an accurate diagnosis. He or she will interview both you and your child. He or she will give your teen a complete physical, psychological, and neurological

exam to rule out physical illness that can look like psychological disturbances, to discover that a "physical" illness is really psychosomatic in
origin, and to determine treatment that will work.

You will find some of the common disorders found in adolescents in
the following chapters. All of the symptoms for these disorders are
based on the diagnoses used in *The Diagnostic and Statistical Manual
of Mental Disorders,* Third Edition, Revised (DSM-III-R). First published in 1980 and updated in 1986–1987, this "psychiatrists' bible" was
designed to help mental health professionals diagnose their patients for
health insurance companies. Although it helps organize the many psychological disorders people have today, it is shrouded in controversy.
Many child psychiatrists have criticized the fact that there has been a
concentration on adult disorders. Others have found it incomplete.
However, the DSM-III-R is the only book to give concise symptoms
for different disorders—but its conclusions are not set in stone. For the
purposes of this book, it's important to keep in mind that the DSM-
III-R is only a tool, not law. Every person is an individual and, as you
look over the symptoms I list for each disorder, remember that they are
generalizations only. Use them for insight, for understanding, and as a
beginning. And always remember to contact your doctor if any of the
symptoms apply to your teen.

In addition to symptoms, I also list unique characteristics and a brief
explanation of available treatments for each disorder.

We have witnessed how children develop. We have seen the ins and
outs of normal adolescence and we have discovered the ways to recognize pain in your teen. Now let's go on—in the following chapters you
will be introduced to the common disorders found in adolescence.

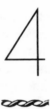

DEPRESSION

Lorna wore a black bandanna in her hair when she was first interviewed at Fair Oaks Hospital. She was neatly groomed but slightly overweight, and her posture was relaxed. Lorna acted like a typical seventeen-year-old teen except for one fact: She smiled and spoke about suicidal thoughts.

Lorna said she'd been depressed for two years, around the time her older brother entered an out-of-state college and she had grown disillusioned with her natural father. Her energy and her school grades subsequently dropped. She began cutting school. She had difficulty concentrating. Five times a week, she drank beer and vodka and she occasionally used marijuana. Two months before she was admitted to Fair Oaks, she had had "scary thoughts" of using a razor to commit suicide: "I'm here because I'm in danger of killing myself and I really do not want to die."

Lorna currently lived in a Pennsylvania suburb with her natural mother, her stepfather, and her sister. Her parents had divorced when she was six and her natural father, at first, lived in a nearby town. Her mother told us that Lorna had appeared to handle the divorce quite well. Though she continued to live with her mother, Lorna saw her natural father frequently. She did not seem to mind when he subsequently remarried and moved to Florida. In fact, until the onset of her depression at fifteen, Lorna was the portrait of a well-adjusted teen. She was an excellent student with no apparent learning disabilities or behavioral problems. She did not have many close friends, but she got along well with others, especially "if they were friendly." Within the family circle, she and her older brother were very close.

But things changed when he went off to college. Lorna suddenly accused her stepfather of "obnoxious pranks": putting soap in her contact lens container, wetting her pillow with water, and stealing her bicycle. She began to withdraw; she got into intense arguments with her mother. Finally, she abruptly told her mother that she was going to live with her natural father in Florida—and moved within two weeks. However, life with father proved to be a disappointment. "He wasn't as warm and understanding as I had thought." Lorna moved back to Pennsylvania after nine months and her depression went from bad to worse.

Lorna had begun to talk to a minister at her church about her suicidal thoughts. He in turn told her mother—who was shocked. She had had no idea that Lorna was so depressed. She brought her to Fair Oaks Hospital in the hope that we would help her get well.

After an extensive examination, we determined that Lorna's depression was the result of a chemical imbalance that had been triggered by past and recent trauma. Though she had appeared to accept her parent's divorce many years ago, she had, in actuality, never expressed her real feelings about it. On one level, there was tremendous guilt and self-loathing. Lorna had subconsciously felt the divorce had been her fault, a just punishment for an oedipal situation that had never been resolved during her childhood development. On another level, there was deep-seated anger and sadness over the past and present losses she had experienced. When her brother went off to school, she felt abandoned—which was compounded by the fact that her natural father, whom she had idealized and who she believed would make everything all right, was only an "ordinary" person. Unable to deal with her inner feelings, she lashed out—at her stepfather. She felt hopeless, helpless, and out of control. Her self-esteem was nil. She knew no way to cope with the stress she was feeling—except through alcohol abuse and suicidal thoughts.

We recommended antidepressant medication, individual, group, and family therapy, antisubstance abuse workshops, assertiveness training, and, to strengthen her self-image, social skills workshops and Performance Group participation. Within six months, Lorna had left the hospital hopeful about her future. She went back to school and she now plans to go on to college. Her depression has abated and the prognosis looks good.

The Symptoms of Depression
Four or more of these symptoms signal depression—and the need for outside help:

- Moody and erratic behavior
- Unhappy and blue feelings
- Irritable and cranky attitudes
- Low self-esteem and guilt
- A lack of enjoyment in previously favorite things
- Death wishes and morbid thoughts
- Withdrawal and loneliness
- Poor or decreased concentration
- Sexual promiscuity and acting out
- Drop in school performance
- Indecisiveness
- Aggressive, petulant, and hostile behavior
- A slowdown in activity level—or a speeded-up hyperactive activity level
- Physical ailments, aches and pains, and general health complaints
- Insomnia—or sleeping too much
- Overeating—or loss of appetite
- Easily tired behavior

The Unique Characteristics of Depression
Depression provides the soil for other disorders. Unable to cope with their feelings of loneliness, fear, anger, and insecurity, many teenagers will turn to self-destructive behavior: substance abuse, delinquency, abusive eating habits, and suicide. They simply don't know any other way to express their pain.

But depression is more than a catalyst to other illnesses. It is also a debilitating disorder all its own. Over 59 percent of all teens who seek out professional help are diagnosed as depressed. But the words "I'm depressed" cover a wide range of depression disorders—all with their different roots, all with their different orientation, and all with their different treatment plans. Teenagers are most susceptible to four kinds of depression. Let's go over each one now.

1. Adjustment Disorder with Depression

Your teen has always been a terrific kid—poised, self-motivated, well-liked, and kind. You were a bit concerned when your company decided to relocate to another state, but you were sure your teen would eventually take it in stride. Wrong. When you mentioned the move, he became withdrawn. His grades dropped. He barely talked to you. And, now that you're in your new home, it's gone from bad to worse. Your once well-adjusted teen has become a sullen, cranky, and sometimes violent stranger.

A new home in a new state. Parents on the verge of divorce. A failing grade on a midterm. Death in the family. All of these situations spell loss and, alone or in combination, they can set an adjustment disorder with depression into motion. Stimulated by external events, this disorder is a teen's attempt to adjust to a life stress that feels overwhelming. It is, pure and simple, a response to loss—both real and imaginary. The danger of this lies in the fact that it is crisis-oriented. Adjustment disorders with depression can come without warning—and lead to drugs, violence, or even suicide before a parent recognizes it for what it is. An adjustment disorder finds fertile soil to grow in any stressful life event, especially:

RELOCATION. Adults know that moving is stressful, almost as stressful, in fact, as divorce or a loved one's death. But its impact on teenagers is sorely underestimated. Moving signifies great loss for teens, not just from leaving a few good friends, but from leaving an entire support system—and an entire world that was comfortable and safe.

RITES OF PASSAGE. Adolescence is filled with chapters that end and new ones that begin. Summer vacation—with its intense, short-lived experiences. A new school term—with its new subjects, teachers, and classmates every fall. High school graduation—with its symbolic embodiment of approaching adulthood. College life—with its pressure-cooker atmosphere of fear and unfamiliarity. Entering the job market—with its rude welcome to the real world of adult responsibility. Rites of passage are a necessary part of growing up, of completion and discovery, but they can also be dangerously stressful transition times of vulnerability and loss.

HURT PRIDE. I remember one of my teenage patients recounting a story about her two best friends. They had decided to drop her because they didn't like her middle name. Another patient told me his girlfriend stopped seeing him because she met someone she thought was "cuter." Life can be cruel to teenagers. From spot quizzes to shallow friendships, from parental judgments to dateless Friday nights—teenagers are constantly being accosted by opportunities for rejection and hurt. And, because they have not yet learned perspective, these painful events can become magnified—and stressful catalysts for depression.

THE SIX STAGES OF ACCEPTANCE

In her landmark book *On Death and Dying* psychiatrist Elisabeth Kübler-Ross outlined six stages patients go through when they discover they have a terminal illness. These same six stages of emotion can apply to any loss—and at any age. A teenager faced with the stress of loss—either through relocation, death, divorce, or rejection—also needs to go through this step-by-step process. In order to cope with the trauma, a teen must move through each one in succession. Problems arise when the teen "gets stuck" in one stage and can't advance to the next. Depression can surface—and the stress from the loss never gets a chance to dissipate. Here are the six stages:

- Denial: "It didn't really happen."
- Anger: "It's not fair!"
- Bargaining: "God, if you take away this pain, I promise I'll be a better person."
- Depression: "I don't want to talk to anyone or do anything. Just leave me alone."
- Acceptance: "It happened and that's that."
- Hope: "It's really going to be okay."

PHYSICAL ILLNESS. Adolescents want and need to be accepted. But a teen who is in and out of hospitals, a teen who has to eat special foods or practice a special routine, a teen who is handicapped by daily insulin shots, a wheelchair, or chronic pain is going to have a more difficult time being accepted than his healthier, untroubled peers. Stress is compounded in physically ill boys when their sexual, athletic, or educational prowess is threatened. Girls feel more stress when their illness makes them feel rejected or isolated. And, regardless of sex, teens with more obvious, severe handicaps will have better self-images than teens with diabetes and other more subtle disabilities. Why? People make more allowances for teens with handicaps that they can see. But teens with more subtle handicaps look normal and are expected to perform as well as others. These factors add pressure to an already stressful situation. In trying to cope, many an ill teen will become overwhelmed—and spiral down into depression.

2. Dysthymia or Chronic Depression

Adjustment disorders with depression are a direct result of external events. But dysthymia has little to do with a teen's outside world. It is an inner war begun long before puberty. Inadequate social or emotional childhood development. Unfinished separation and individuation between parent and child. Cognitive growth impairment. An improperly developed self-identity. Any of these can result in dysthymia. In fact, a 1967 study by Dr. Sandor Lorand found that teens who craved reassurance and love had not been adequately nourished during childhood development. Instead, their pain and anxiety was internalized, creating feelings of low self-esteem, pessimism, and hopelessness that stayed with them as they grew.

Chronically depressed teens are indeed their "own worst enemy." Listen to one of the members of the Fair Oaks Hospital Performance Group: "I understand the fact that I create most of my problems. But changing will be difficult and slow. That's because talking like this to a group of people about my weaknesses and faults is new and frightening. Also feeling happy and accepted and good about myself is a feeling that I'm unaccustomed to." Life is a difficult, gray, and unyielding road for the dysthymic teen. Here are some of the reasons why dysthymia is so insidious:

A NEGATIVE OUTLOOK ON LIFE. Helpless and hopeless are the bylaws of the chronically depressed teen. As Dr. Meeks says in *High Times/Low Times,* "They are true pessimists, always expecting the worst, which, more times than not, becomes a self-fulfilling prophecy." When Dr. Daniel Offer surveyed chronically depressed teens, he found that they had problems with their feelings and their relationships with family and friends. They were not able to cope well with stress and they were overly concerned with what others thought of them. They felt unattractive. Their self-esteem was nil and they did not feel good about themselves. This inner turmoil leads to poor concentration, low energy, and sleep and appetite disturbances.

A PERVASIVE FEELING OF POWERLESSNESS. Dysthymic teens never feel that their actions have an impact on the world. They can never change things—or change the way they feel. They simply close their minds to good news; they are terrified it will only get snatched away. Similarly, they will avoid encouragement and support. "I'll only be let down," said one dysthymic teen. These teens feel like victims of the "terrible" world around them. But, in reality, they are victims of their own fate—because they feel so powerless to change.

AN INABILITY TO EXPRESS ANGER. Dysthymic teens live in a war-torn battlefield filled with conflicting emotions and uncertainty. Because they care so much about other people's opinions, they can never speak their minds. Because they can never be sure their emotions are valid, they will try to hide the way they feel. Because they are terrified that their emotions, once unleashed, will get out of control, they can never get angry—or confront anyone or anything head-on. These inner, emotional struggles are complicated by the fact that dysthymic teens have high morals and an overriding sense of right and wrong. For them, as Daniel Offer's study also discovered, self-destructive behavior comes not from a renunciation of the world—but from a perceived inability to live up to its standards.

LOW SELF-ESTEEM. In 1969 Drs. Ruth K. Goldman and Gerald A. Mendelsohn surveyed psychotherapists across the country to discover what they considered the most important aspect of mental health. The overwhelming answer? A positive self-image. In chapter one, we have seen how important and far-reaching the development of the self is in childhood. A child whose self-esteem is stymied in the early developmental years will be left with a nagging emptiness and insecurity, a pervasive feeling that she doesn't measure up to her parents' expectations. When the developmental process is repeated in adolescence, she will continue to hate herself—but on a larger scale. As a teenager, she not only doesn't measure up at home—but also at school and among her peers. The result is instability—and a chronic depressed view of herself and her place in the world.

3. Major Depression: Single Episode or Recurrent

Delia, a patient at Fair Oaks, had been diagnosed with a rare blood disease when she was only nine years old. She spent the next several years in and out of hospitals, isolated from others, and, when she turned fifteen, she tried to kill herself with an overdose of penicillin tablets.

A major depression can be triggered by stress in a predisposed and susceptible teen. In Delia's case, it was susceptibility. Years and years of stress from her physical illness made her vulnerable. When she was hospitalized yet again for her condition at fifteen, the hospitalization was "the last straw." Combined with ongoing family problems, the incident overwhelmed her. Delia couldn't fathom any other way to cope—except suicide.

THE MANY MASKS OF DEPRESSION

Sometimes a depression doesn't look like one. Instead of withdrawal, moodiness, rebellion, and tears, your teen might develop physical pain: backaches, stomachaches, headaches, dizziness, palpitations, tingly sensations in her fingers and toes, and more. This is called a *masked depression.* Though the physical pains are real, your teen's aches and pains are, in actuality, an expression of her mental anguish.

Only your physician can determine whether your teen is in fact physically ill or depressed, but here's a clue: If your teen gets a clean bill of health from her doctor but refuses to believe it, the chances are good that she is suffering from depression.

Most major depressions are endogenous, which means, literally, "from within." Triggered by stress, a chemical imbalance occurs in the brain and a teen becomes depressed.

4. Bipolar Disorder

Margaret had always been a quiet, shy child. But when she entered high school, she became even more withdrawn. Her grades, energy, and concentration dropped. She began to lose weight; she had trouble sleeping. Her maternal grandmother had been depressed when she was younger and her mother, recognizing the signs, took Margaret to a psychiatrist. She was diagnosed as having a major depression. With medication and therapy, Margaret seemed to to get better. But two years later, she developed a different modus operandi. She started dressing very provocatively. She stayed up for nights on end. She began squandering all her allowance on "punk" clothes and she began babbling about writing the great American novel. Unfortunately, Margaret's parents accredited her new behavior to rebellion. They didn't make any link between Margaret's major depression two years ago and her manic behavior today.

Manic-depressive episodes don't happen only to adults. Many teens suffer from this same disorder—but they elude diagnosis. The true definition of Bipolar Disorders, according to Dr. Gabrielle A. Carlson, writing in the *Psychiatric Annals,* are "very clear-cut depressive episodes followed by a manic episode." Margaret's so-called major depression two years ago was, in actuality, a depressive episode in the bipolar disorder cycle.

Margaret's misdiagnosis is more common than you might think. Many bipolar disorders have been called adjustment disorders or major depressions because the first depressive episode occurred after a stressful event. But a manic stage will always appear in time. In fact, a study of adolescents hospitalized for depression found that 20 percent of them had a manic episode within three years after their discharge.

As we have seen in chapter two, most teenagers go through their adolescence with little difficulty. Not every teen develops one of these depressive disorders. But there are eight kinds of adolescents who are more susceptible to depression. Let's examine more closely those at risk:

OVERACHIEVERS. Adolescent psychiatrist John E. Meeks calls them "Type A" kids: teenagers who are driven to succeed—with no room for failure. Like their adult counterparts, these teens are bright, charming, and energetic. But underneath this charismatic persona lies a very fragile identity, one that is ready to crumble at the slightest provocation. The only way "Type A" teens can build up their low self-esteem is through outside achievement. Good grades, lots of friends, student leadership positions—all validate their success as people, all keep insecurity and fear at bay. But perfection is impossible to maintain—and "Type A" teens know that better than anyone. Anxiety builds and eventually their worst fears come true. They get a lower grade on a test. They have a fight with a friend. They overhear an insensitive remark. Depression sets in and the world of the overachiever will start to crumble. Unfortunately, adults don't always recognize the "Type A" kid's need for support and help. Because they seem so self-confident, these teens often suffer in silence, boxed in a corner, with only one perceived way out: suicide.

CHILDREN OF DYSFUNCTIONAL FAMILIES. "All happy families are like one another; each unhappy family is unhappy in its own way." When Leo Tolstoy wrote these words in *Anna Karenina,* he was talking about the individual dramas that are played out in unhappy family circles. But what is not unique in unhappy families is the legacy of pain that is passed down from generation to generation. A study of over 1,200 Australian adolescents found that depression was three times more prevalent in teens who did not feel they had a close or loving family relationship. Another study, conducted by the pioneering adolescent psychiatrist Dr. Michael Rutter, analyzed 137 children of 43 depressed parents. His results? Nearly 50 percent of these children had a diagnosable psychiatric disorder. In study after study, the evidence is clear: a dysfunctional family atmosphere will make a child more susceptible to depression.

On the other hand, a healthy family environment will foster healthy adolescent development. A study of adolescent boys found that mothers with high self-esteem had sons with high self-esteem—and there was little parental conflict or marital discord within the family circle.

PESSIMISTIC TEENS. An infant will internalize whatever he sees reflected on his mother's face. Dr. Heinz Kohut called this process "mirroring"—and it is an important factor in healthy self-development. If his mother is smiling, he will feel good. But if she is depressed and sullen, her dour demeanor will be reflected onto him—and he will develop a sense of unworthiness and pessimism. By the time he reaches adolescence, his pessimism is intact—and, cognitively, he can only think of himself as that unworthy infant. The "mirrors" he looks at in the outside world can only reflect and reinforce his hopeless and helpless view of life.

There is also an element of fear in pessimistic teens. They are usually extremely sensitive, responding so intensely to stimuli that they learn to fear their actions—and the "horrible" world around them.

You can recognize a pessimistic teen from his aura of despair: a sloppy, unkempt appearance, an uncommunicative, sluggish demeanor, and a sullen, downcast face.

LEARNING-DISABLED TEENS. Like the chicken or the egg, it's difficult to always know which came first: the learning disability or the depression. The depressive disorder can be the result of a chemical imbalance that was there long before the learning disability was ever diagnosed—or a learning disability can cause the stress that makes a teen depressed.

Take the example of Allen, a young boy with dyslexia. Before his dyslexia was discovered, he appeared to be a well-adjusted eleven-year-old. He went to school every day and, like his other classmates, tried to participate in class. But he fell further and further behind in his assignments; he simply couldn't keep up. He grew frustrated because he couldn't understand. This frustration led to boredom—which led to depression. Soon Allen was acting out in class; his teachers branded him a troublemaker. By the time his dyslexia was diagnosed, it was almost too late. Allen had already learned to feel like a "loser." He no longer had the inclination to do his schoolwork. He stopped trying to succeed.

In today's world, Allen's story might have a happier ending. Parents and teachers are recognizing learning disabilities at an earlier age. But a child who reaches adolescence with an undisclosed—or ignored—learning disability usually has two problems to overcome: the disability and the depression. And it doesn't matter whether it was "the chicken or the egg" that came first.

CONDUCT-DISORDERED TEENS. Here's an excerpt from an interview I had with Bill, a sixteen-year-old patient at Fair Oaks Hospital:

> **DR. R:** What do you get out of stealing? Why do you like it so much?
> **BILL:** It's just different. I've done stupid things. There was a hot-dog stand. I broke into it. I didn't take the money. I took three cases of hot-dog buns.
> **DR. R:** And what did you do with them?
> **BILL:** I just had them. I did it. I wound up giving them away.
> **DR. R:** So there's something exciting about the whole idea of stealing, of checking the place out, of finally getting in there. That's exciting to you. That's what you like?
> **BILL:** Yeah.

Bill has a conduct disorder. Like many other teenagers, he has translated his fear of dependency, his low self-esteem, and his inability to cope with the unknown, outside world into self-destructive action. Rather than confront his "embarrassing" needs and vulnerability, he acts tough. But just below the surface lies depression—and an unyielding, primitive conscience. Conduct-disordered teens usually come from homes where punishment is arbitrary and severe. Reasoning and discussion are nil: "You'll do what I say—or else!" Consequently, their moral development is stymied. Instead of a moral system based on an inner sense of right and wrong, they develop one of built of external, black-and-white rigidity. As they approach adolescence, their new emotions and impulses can find no acceptable outlet. Guilt-ridden, ashamed, and fearful of reprisal, these teens can express themselves only through hell-bent, unthinking self-destruction. They stay one step ahead of their depression with excitement—in the form of drug addiction, stealing, sexual promiscuity, and violence.

OVERPROTECTED ADOLESCENTS. Too much love can be as bad as too little. Sometimes the problem begins during the separation and individuation stages of childhood development. Overly protective parents won't allow their toddler to crawl away and explore—or they will watch him with anxious eyes. Their anxiety is transferred to the child; he becomes overly dependent and fearful of the world. Sometimes, however, it's simply a case of too much of a good thing. Consider Arlene, a child loved and adored by her parents. Because they had her late in life, they doted on her; she was the most beautiful, talented, and brilliant girl ever born. But when Arlene became an adolescent, she found that the high self-esteem she had developed as a child had no place to develop in the real world. Her grades were only average. The boys did not line up at her door. Her writing, artwork, and piano playing were mediocre. Without any positive feedback from the outside world, she fell back on her parents—where she could be assured of security and esteem. But there was a price. Instead of developing independence, Arlene developed stagnation. She began to resent her parents; they had lied to her. But she felt too guilt-ridden and scared to vocalize her pain. Instead, Arlene said nothing. But, inside, her emotions were dancing out of control. Her parents' loving but overprotective stance became an unintentional route to depression.

LONERS. Hamilton came to Fair Oaks Hospital's Adolescent Unit with the steadfast belief that television transmitters were watching him night and day. Carmine imagined she had become president of the United States without ever running for office. Samantha refused to acknowledge that her stuffed animal was only a toy. Schizophrenia is a biological disorder, a direct result of a chemical imbalance in the brain. Only 1 percent of the general population is diagnosed as schizophrenic, and onset begins in adolescence.

Not every loner becomes a schizophrenic, but a teen is susceptible if he:

- Has a family history of schizophrenia
- Lives in an unreal fantasy world
- Forms unrealistic goals and never pursues them
- Displays symptoms of depression or antisocial behavior
- Lacks the skills to cope with stress
- Constantly blames outside "demons" instead of confronting the changes going on within himself.

ABUSED TEENS. From the headlines in today's papers to television's "docudrama" movies, sexual and physical abuse has become a cause célèbre, a terrible and unfortunate reality of American family life. Some facts:

- Over 2 million children were abused in 1986—30 percent of them physically abused and almost 55 percent of them neglected.
- Over 130,000 youngsters are sexually abused every year.
- Nearly 1,300 letters received by *Glamour* magazine in a recent survey by Leslie Dormen on sexual abuse were from women who were victims of sexual abuse before they reached eighteen.

Abuse can be sexual or physical—or a condition of emotional neglect. It is more than an isolated stressful event. It is a situation with aftershocks that reverberate in its victims well into adulthood. Fear of physical contact, promiscuity, guilt, shame, and depression—all can be a direct result of an earlier abuse. Today, more and more adolescents are encouraged to talk about their abuse, but many cases still stay under wraps. Unfortunately, this keeps the myth of "It was all my fault" alive. Worse, when these children become parents themselves, statistics show they can continue the abuse they learned at home—and abuse their own children.

Treating Depression
Substance abuse . . . eating disorders . . . anxiety disorders . . . learning disabilities . . . conduct disorders. In the next several chapters, you will be reading about other common adolescent disorders—all of which are combined with depression. And, in order to treat each of them successfully, you must also treat the underlying depression. But treating depression is a multifaceted task. Major depressions and bipolar disorders are usually triggered by a chemical imbalance and require antidepressant medication. Adjustment disorders with depression and dysthymia

may or may not be biologically based. All of these depressions, however, require therapy—both in treating the symptoms of depression and in treating the way a teen copes with stress. If the stress a teen experiences through loss, physical illness, or rejection is not addressed, the depression can return.

When I first see a new patient and his family, I record what I call the teen's "lifeline"—an extensive history of stressful life events he has experienced throughout all his developmental stages. This lifeline helps me determine the traumas a teen faced during his childhood development, the traumas he is experiencing now as a developing adolescent, the potential traumas he might face as an adult, and the way he has perceived his stressful life events throughout the years. All these factors must be combined in a successful treatment plan, and I will be discussing the specific medications and types of therapies available today in later chapters.

ARE YOU DEPRESSED?

Depressed parents can pass their illness on to their children. If any of these statements sound familiar, you would be wise to seek outside professional help. Depression in adults, as in teens, can be treated successfully—as long as it is not ignored.

1. I sometimes feel as if everybody's against me.
2. I've lost my appetite—or I can't seem to stop eating.
3. I hate my looks.
4. I have trouble sleeping.
5. I've become a real "couch potato."
6. I've lost my desire for sex.
7. Everything takes so much effort—even going to the supermarket is too much of a chore.
8. I started to drink in the afternoon.
9. I'm really worried about my health.
10. I don't feel like seeing my friends.
11. I can't seem to do anything right.
12. I start crying for no reason.
13. I haven't taken a shower in days—and I don't care.
14. I feel as if I'm all alone.
15. Life is dull.

Depression is a complicated disease, with many unique variables that come into play. It can follow a stressful event without any rhyme or reason. It can come to roost when a family history of depression is present. And it may or may not strike a biochemically susceptible teen. Only a professional can determine whether depression is present. But only you, the parent, can determine whether a problem is present in the first place—by understanding and watching for the warning signs.

Depression can be cured—as long as it is not ignored or minimized. Fear can become hope. Rejection can become acceptance. Insecurity can become self-confidence. As a teenager in a Performance Group audience once said, "I can finally see the light at the end of the tunnel. It is possible to be happy."

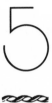

5

SUBSTANCE ABUSE

"I'm only here for an evaluation." That's Brenda talking, ready to leap off her chair and out the door of the Fair Oaks Hospital's admissions office. We could barely hear her responses to the questions we asked; she was angry, hostile, and frightened. Brenda started smoking cigarettes when she was nine years old. She began to drink and smoke marijuana in sixth grade. By the time she was twelve, she had used PCP, LSD, mescaline, cocaine, amphetamines, Valium, and had inhaled lighter fluid from cigarette lighters. That was two years ago. On this day, in the admissions office, she was barely fourteen.

Brenda lived with her mother, father, and younger sister in New York State. She had been hospitalized four times in the past three years and Fair Oaks was her parents' last hope. "Home," her mother said, "had become a nightmare." Brenda drinking. Brenda hitting her sister. Brenda screaming at her parents. Brenda cutting her arms and legs with disposable razors.

When we asked her about these accusations, Brenda shrugged. "I hate them and they hate me." She was angry with them because they wouldn't let her "party with her friends or even be alone in the house."

Brenda was a troubled teen. But, on the surface, she looked as if the world could be hers for the asking. Tall and slender, with blond hair and blue eyes, she had the demeanor of a fashion model. She was well-groomed and dressed in the latest style. But her stance was defensive; she was fidgety. She had an aura of vulnerability beneath her hostility. In the past, her doctors diagnosed her as having neurological disorders, learning disabilities, aberrant personality disorders, and conduct disorders. Her previous hospitalizations were failures. Her substance abuse and self-destructive behavior continued—and grew worse.

Her parents described Brenda as a "delightful child." Until she was ten years old, her grades were excellent; she had many friends. But today was a different story. Their child had become a terrifying stranger. She was failing at school. She had lost weight. She couldn't sleep. She was out of control.

The past held clues to her present behavior. Brenda's father had been diagnosed as clinically depressed; he had been out of work for over two years around the time Brenda had begun "acting out." Money grew tight. He and Brenda's mother separated for a few months. When he returned to the house, they continued to battle with each other. Lately, their fights were over Brenda.

When we tested her, we could find nothing physiologically abnormal; she was a healthy teenaged girl. Despite the previous litany of diagnoses, we recognized that Brenda was suffering from recurrent major depression, which had found a destructive outlet in drugs. Brenda had family problems; the dysfunctional family atmosphere hindered her emotional and social development. The discord at home was a stress she couldn't handle. Her low self-esteem, her fears, her hopeless stance were all compounded by her inability to cope.

At Fair Oaks, she was put on medication to help her depression. She participated in anti-substance-abuse workshops. She was involved in individual, group, and family therapy. After seven months, Brenda was ready to go home. She was off drugs—and had no desire to go back to them. She had gained insight into her family problems. She had learned new coping skills and she no longer hated herself or her life.

Today, Brenda is still drug-free. She sees a therapist once a week. Her parents have divorced. Brenda lives with her mother and home has become a calmer place. She plans on studying fashion when she finishes high school. Someday she'd like to own her own clothing boutique.

The Symptoms of Substance Abuse
One or more of these symptoms can mean possible alcohol or drug abuse in your teen:

- Physical evidence of drugs and related paraphernalia
- Loss of appetite
- Inability to have fun
- Red or dilated eyes
- Enjoyable activities dropped—with nothing to replace them
- Few interests or hobbies
- Hostile, dishonest, and manipulative relationships with others
- Irritable and erratic behavior
- Irresponsibility
- Sniffling, runny nose
- Anger and raised voices to parents
- Self-neglect
- Withdrawal from friends and family
- Loss of money and valuables around the house
- Diminished memory
- Drop in school grades and truancy
- Chronic lying
- Change of friends
- Parents' "gut" feeling that their teen has become a stranger

There is one symptom of substance abuse that is not on this list. It is a condition that can discount all these other signs—and make a drug problem worse. It's called *denial.*

No one in the family is immune to its call—not parents and not the drug-abusing teens themselves. "The primary factors interfering with the diagnosis of chemical dependency in adolescence," writes Robert Lee Hendren in the American Psychiatric Association's *Annual Review,* "are the patient's and the family's tendencies to deny the illness."

It makes sense. No one likes to admit they have a problem, especially a teenager who is struggling with conflicting and confusing emotions. Many teens turn to drugs because of this inner turmoil. How can they turn around and say the one thing that has kept their inner "demons" at bay is really a sham? How can they admit that they've become dependent on the one thing they found to *avoid* dependency? To renounce drugs would mean facing, in their minds, a terrifying, pain-filled void. In fact, the more addicted the teen, the greater the anxiety—and the greater the denial. "It's no problem. I can quit anytime" is said as much for their parent's benefit as for their own. A study of 189 addicted adolescents bears this out: 89 percent of the adolescents reported using alcohol, but only 25 percent said they had a problem with it. And, the more addicted they were, the stronger was their disclaimer.

There was another result of that same study—and it had to do with the mothers of the addicted teens. The mothers, when interviewed, knew their kids drank alcohol—but they had had no idea that they also used tranquilizers, barbiturates, sedatives, and other drugs. These mothers are not alone. I have seen parents who've walked past their teenager's closed door for months, the cloying smell of marijuana wafting through the cracks, only to open a window because "It's really stuffy in here." I have seen drug paraphernalia come tumbling out of a teenager's pocketbook at her parents' feet—and they never even noticed. I had a teenager tell me that he was "stoned out of his head all of the time for years"—without his parents saying a word. The fact is that parents are as guilty of denial as their children. Most families don't adapt well to change. They'd rather sweep things under the rug than confront a problem that is so painful, so complex, and so stressful that it could very well change the family balance forever. Embarrassment, fear, guilt—all play their role in a family's denial.

Whether it's done in the name of love or out of fear or ignorance, denial simply enables an addiction to continue—and get worse. But to be forearmed is to be forewarned. Parents owe it to their children and to themselves to observe and watch—and to intervene at the slightest indication of substance abuse.

The Unique Characteristics of Substance Abuse

- One out of every fifty high school seniors smokes marijuana every day.
- 41 percent of all high school seniors have tried smoking marijuana at least once.
- 29 percent of high school seniors nationwide have tried drugs other than marijuana.
- 32 percent of all high school seniors have had, by their own admission, five or more drinks in a row within the last thirty days.
- Alcohol and drug abuse costs our society $205 billion every year.
- Although 91 percent of all high school seniors acknowledge that regular use of cocaine is dangerous, only 59 percent saw much risk in trying it.

Drugs seduce. Period. Despite the success of America's "Just Say No" campaign, despite the bad publicity given drugs like crack and cocaine, despite all the facts and all the figures, teens are continuing to do drugs—many of them before they even reach junior high. As one of my former patients recently told me during a follow-up interview: "I'm really glad I'm off drugs and I'll never go back. But nothing will ever equal the high I got from cocaine."

Unfortunately, it's this "high" that first tempts teenagers—without regard for the equally high price that drugs extract. Teenagers are, on the whole, impulsive and action-oriented. They can't put things into perspective—especially a future that seems limitless. Educators are becoming aware of this. Antismoking classes for teenagers now stress bad breath and odor instead of lung cancer and emphysema.

Seduction weaves a powerful web, but there are three other reasons why teens take drugs:

1. Drugs: The "Adult" Way to Cope

Teenagers struggle to grow up. As we have seen, their development can be fraught with anxiety—socially, emotionally, and cognitively. They see adults using cigarettes, alcohol, and other drugs to relieve their tension. So why can't they use drugs, too? Drugs become a symbol of the adult world—with the added plus of keeping their anxiety at bay. Studies show that if parents smoke or drink, chances are greater that their children will also pick up the habit—especially if the parents have permissive attitudes.

THE FOUR STEPS TO TEENAGE ADDICTION

Full-blown addictions don't happen overnight. They occur in stages. Recognizing these steps can help you act early to prevent a problem later:

1. Experimentation. This is the "tryout" stage where, because of peer pressure, a teen might try a can of beer or a joint. The euphoria he feels is quickly dissipated, and he will soon return to normal. But he remembers the pleasant feeling—and may come back for more.

2. Social-Recreational Use. An occasional use becomes more regular use—maybe on school nights, maybe a few times during the week. Teens start to miss the "high" when they don't have it. Symptoms of drug abuse will start cropping up.

3. Preoccupation. It's now an obsession—and definitely more than that occasional beer. Teens at this stage probably are using more and more illegal drugs. They've missed school. They've dropped their "straight" friends. They begin to steal for their habit.

4. Dependency. Addiction is now a reality—and the teen can no longer see things clearly. The drugs are in control and he must get help before it is too late.

A study of 654 teenagers by Michael D. Newcomb and P. M. Bentler brings this adult point of view home in a surprising way. When these teenagers drank, it actually had some positive effects on their self-esteem, their relationships with their families, and in romantic social situations—just as it can for adults. Why? Because alcohol is not illegal in the adult world, and it doesn't have as much of a negative connotation as other drugs. A teenager's parents will condone alcohol consumption more readily—especially if the choice is between alcohol and other drugs. And, because alcohol reduces inhibitions, a drink can make a teen feel less awkward socially.

But the researchers caution that alcohol use does not mean misuse. A teenaged boy who had been at Fair Oaks Hospital for drug and alcohol abuse had come back a second time. He was perplexed that his parents made him go back to the hospital. "I started drinking again, but I didn't take any street drugs." After he was released a second time, he now knows that alcohol can be an insidious drug all on its own—and just as addicting as illegal substances. As Dr. Dorynne Czechowicz wrote in the *American Journal of Drug and Alcohol Abuse,* "Alcohol-related traffic accidents kill 8,000 persons 15–24 years of age each year—the leading cause of death in this age group."

Drugs might symbolize the adult world teenagers are struggling toward, but they also provide a means of controlling their need to be children, to depend on their parents for love and support. Drugs give them distance and allow them to stay "one step away" from their fears. Unfortunately, this control is a house of cards. Without inner growth, it will fall apart.

2. Drugs and Peer Pressure

Teens want to belong. If "everybody's doing it," they'll be hard-pressed to join in. And, the more they say "no," the more pressure they will receive from their peers. A study of adolescent drinking by Dr. Robert W. Conroy found that alcohol consumption was directly related to the number of friends who drink, the amount these friends drink, and whether or not these friends approved of drinking. Another study found that 30 percent of all high school students were pressured by their friends, at one time or another, to have a cigarette or a drink.

Teens also have a tendency to exaggerate—and that includes drugs and alcohol. When someone tells a teen, "I don't know a person who hasn't tried it," the teen truly believes it. Add the "fun" factor—and the pressure is increased tenfold. As one study showed, most teens who use marijuana say they do so because "it feels good."

"Just Say No" is difficult—but it's not impossible. If a teenager has strong religious and family ties the chances are great that he or she will not succumb to peer pressure—regardless of how "good" it feels to belong.

3. Drugs Mask Depression

Depression hurts. In chapter four, we explored the effects of lonely, frustrated, and angry feelings. If a teenager cannot cope with the stress of adolescent life, he or she will do what his parents might do: self-medicate. As Sandra Gardner wrote in the book *Teenage Suicide:*

Feelings are painful, and the teenager feels helpless about doing anything about the problems causing the pain. He doesn't think he has permission to express these feelings. He may be laughed at. His parents may think he's making a big deal out of nothing. His friends might not understand. His parents may be so wrapped up in their own problems that he perceives he can't burden them with his.

Instead, a depressed teen will turn to alcohol and drugs. As in the case study of Brenda at the beginning of this chapter, this drug experimentation leads to abuse—and the slow, torturous road to self-destruction.

Here's more proof: Low self-esteem, depression, and anxiety were all found in adolescents who abused drugs in rural populations. And, in a study in 1980 by Dr. Howard B. Kaplan, low self-esteem was found to predispose teenagers to use alcohol, marijuana, and narcotics.

In fact, depression is the most insidious reason teenagers use drugs. Masking pain with a "quick fix" is only temporary at best—and addictive at worst. The more teens take drugs to mask their pain, the more their tolerance builds—and the more they need to get "high." But these higher dosages mean more harmful side effects—both physically and psychologically.

Simply trying a drug does not mean addiction. A healthy teen will stop if he or she:

- Finds parental disapproval
- Can't readily get any more
- Has a minor brush with the law
- Recognizes that the drug is interfering with long-range plans and goals

But why do some teenagers get trapped on this destructive roller-coaster ride—and others don't? There are many reasons for teenage addiction, including:

The drugs of first choice are adult drugs—which are more likely to lead to abuse. The girl wears a tasteful, but clingy, black dress. Her ears, neck, and wrists drip with diamonds. She points her beautifully made-up face at an equally beautiful man—who sports a winter tan and an elegant black tuxedo. This is not a scene from a 1940s melodrama. Nor is it an excerpt from a recent "Lifestyles of the Rich and Famous." It is a generic magazine ad, selling cigarettes or liquor to susceptible teens. As we have seen, "adult" drugs symbolize an adult world that both attracts and repels adolescents. Cigarettes and alcohol are not only a part of that brave new world, they are also legal and easily available. Studies show that if a teen smokes or drinks, the chances are good that he will not only try an illegal drug—but abuse it.

CIGARETTE SMOKING IS HARMFUL TO YOUR TEEN'S HEALTH

- 90 percent of adult smokers started before the age of nineteen.
- One out of every five high school seniors smoke cigarettes on a daily basis—and more girls smoke than boys.
- Teenaged girls who smoke cigarettes are more likely to to move on to other drugs.
- Teenagers who start smoking in early adolescence have a greater chance of developing physical ailments, emotional distress, problems with social relationships, and some form of family strife by the time they reach late adolescence.

Teens are more vulnerable than adults to drugs. Adults need between four and five years to become addicts—but teenagers need only fifteen and a half months. Teenagers are still developing. Their minds and bodies have not yet matured. If teens begin to take drugs, they probably aren't getting enough sleep or proper nutrition. This keeps their bodies soft and leads to poor concentration, memory lapses, and lethargy. They soon lose interest in the world around them, and their drugs become their only "anchor." In order to control their increasing confusion, they cling to their drugs, and addiction begins to accelerate.

The fact that the drugs found on the streets today are more potent and dangerous than those sold only twenty years ago makes this process even more insidious. Here are some examples:

- *Crack* is an inexpensive, readily available form of cocaine that causes addiction within three or four *weeks* of experimentation. Like heroin, its initial rush is so intense that people prefer to use it in solitude.
- *Cocaine* and *speed* are stimulants that lead to severe withdrawal and physiological depression. At first, although energy seems to increase, lethargy, paranoia, and depression will eventually set in—as will mucus membrane damage.
- *Marijuana, alcohol,* and *"downers"* are depressants that go to work immediately on the central nervous system, producing an emotional and biochemical depressive reaction. Initially, there's a euphoric feeling of relief as the drug raises the body's blood level— only to dissipate into depression as the drug begins to wear off.

- *PCP—phencyclidine* or *angel dust*—promotes hallucinogenic, psychotic behavior. Teens on PCP can be dangerous—both to others and to themselves. They will act impulsively and violently. Angel dust can also cause numbness.
- *Minor tranquilizers* were created to save lives, but, unfortunately, they too can be abused. Teens often take them in dangerous combinations with other drugs. When Valium, for example, is combined with alcohol, it can produce a coma. Antidepressants are the most common drugs used in teenage suicides—which is why they must be carefully monitored when used in the therapeutic process.

Antisocial activities lead teens to drugs—which encourage more antisocial actions. A ten-year study of urban black first-grade students found that those who were aggressive did drugs on a regular basis by the tenth grade. A five-to-nine-year study of male criminals discovered that men who abused drugs since the ninth grade had twice as many traffic violations, property damage violations, and drug-related arrests than those who didn't. Here's another scenario: A quiet, unaggressive teenager starts doing drugs and becomes addicted. Suddenly, he needs money for his habit and he begins to do things that he'd never dreamed of doing—stealing money out of his mother's purse, stealing his father's watch, robbing a corner store. The guilt from these actions makes him depressed. To keep his pain away, he needs more drugs—and he'll commit more antisocial acts to get them.

The drug scene is secretive, manipulative, and deceitful. The world of illegal drugs is not known for its nurturing atmosphere. In fact, the more involved a teen becomes in her habit, the more the drug environment destroys the supportive, caring relationships that were once a part of her world. Without her parents, other adults, or her "straight" friends to rely on, she depends more and more on her drugs—and moves farther along the road to addiction. As a former Performance Group member once told a teenage audience: "When I was coming down from being high, I felt like I didn't deserve anything except to get high again because it made me feel good about myself. But in the meantime I had lost my straight friends and that made me feel even more insecure. I felt really rejected . . . drugs were the answer to make me feel better."

Addiction is hereditary. One of the ten risks of coronary heart disease is a family history of heart attacks. Similarly, if someone in your family is an addict, the risk is greater that you—or your children—will become one as well. Studies of identical twins found that if one twin was an addict, there was a 54 percent chance of the other twin becoming one. A landmark study done in Denmark on adoption showed that adopted sons have a four to five times greater risk of being an alcoholic if their natural father was one—even if they never knew him or lived with him. Nowhere is the hereditary factor more telling or sad than in the recent epidemic of "crack" babies. Because their mothers used crack during their pregnancy, these babies were born addicted.

Sometimes, however, it's not the addiction that's inherited, but a sensitivity to chemicals. In 1985 Drs. Douglas R. Robbins and Norman E. Alessi found that people with depression disorders had this sensitivity—which was combined with a limited tolerance. Because of their depression, many of these chemically sensitive teens can be drawn to drugs—only to find that their low tolerance level turns them into addicts.

Addictive behavior can begin at home. Picture this scenario: Your father comes home from work and immediately makes himself a scotch on the rocks. He sits down and relaxes with one more before dinner. Your mother joins him with a glass of white wine and a cigarette. You, the thirteen-year-old teenager, can only watch, attempting to do your homework—but all the while, you're wishing you were already an adult so you could join the fun. Studies show that you'd be a prime candidate for addiction, following the same patterns as your parents.

As we have seen, the environment can play as large a role as heredity in childhood and adolescent development. It can also play as large a role in addiction. A study of over 1,200 high school students found that alcohol, cigarette, and marijuana consumption was twice as high in teens who had family difficulties as in teens who had nurturing homes. Another study found that addicted adolescent girls felt they had a poor relationship with their mothers—especially if they were raised in single-parent households. And yet another study, this time of eight hundred adolescents, found that when the father was absent from the home, there was a greater use of alcohol and marijuana—particularly in boys.

Other environmental factors include:

- Socioeconomic class
- Ethnic and religious background
- Drug availability
- Drug-taking frequency
- Past developmental history

The reasons why some teens become addicted vary from individual to individual. Genetics. Family life. Antisocial behavior. The list goes on. But the main theme linking all the different variables is: *When drugs become more important than interacting with others, a teen becomes chemically addicted.* As a Fair Oaks Hospital patient wrote to her brother: "Why did you ruin your life with drugs and alcohol? I know that you struggle. So do I. But why couldn't you have dealt with your sadness? When all you were doing was ruining your life. And I know you know."

Understand. Observe. And intervene. Substance abuse *can* be prevented.

Treating Substance Abuse

So far, this chapter has been full of information about bad things that can happen to teenagers. The good news is that teenagers are highly resilient. Because they are young, they bounce back quickly. And, because they haven't been on drugs as long as their adult counterparts, their withdrawal symptoms won't be as severe.

Treatment can begin only with total abstinence. If an addicted teen could smoke one joint and put it out for good, he wouldn't be an addict. The fact is that teenagers who are still taking drugs, no matter how small the dosage, will continue to deny their problems—and never be helped. As an added plus, stopping becomes its own motivation. As a teen comes out of her "drug-induced cloud," she begins to feel better; she feels a sense of relief which helps abstinence continue. Further, because hospitals can supply a safe environment of total abstinence, most substance abuse programs require at least a short-term hospital stay. A hospital can also supply medical supervision of withdrawal stages.

As reported by Dr. Dorynne Czechowicz in the *American Journal of Drug and Alcohol Abuse,* a recent study from the National Institute of Mental Health showed that prompt identification and treatment of preexisting and/or coexisting mental illness could prevent a significant amount of drug abuse. At Fair Oaks Hospital, we believe in treating this underlying depression or conduct disorder as well as the substance abuse problem. We also want our teens to gain insight as to why they chose drugs—and what choices would be more appropriate and healthier to opt for in the future. To that end, as with depression, we construct a patient lifeline to determine past and present stress—and we concentrate our therapeutic efforts on teaching the teens to understand and cope with stress in better, more productive ways.

Though Alcoholics Anonymous–like treatment plans are popular today, it is my belief that the "12 Steps" method doesn't work as well with adolescents. Teenagers are still developing; they are not yet emotionally or morally mature enough to "give up control" to the group. Instead, I stress the importance of knowing how a teen got to the hospital—giving him a chance to look at his strengths and weaknesses, his problems and solutions, and, hopefully, to discover eventually that he *does* have some control over his life. I do, however, encourage our patients to join AA and Narcotics Anonymous—but only as a network of support, a way to meet peers in the same position as themselves.

There is one area where all substance abuse programs are in agreement: the very real need for communication between family members in substance abuse disorders. Family therapy is crucial. As one study discovered, many adolescents minimize their drug problem and exaggerate the family discord at home. Their parents, on the other hand, claim that their teen's drug problem is the culprit—destroying what would otherwise be a perfectly fine family environment.

Within the entire therapeutic process, there is always the danger that addicted teens will have a relapse. They might forget they had had a drug problem—and start the denial process. They might yearn for drugs during a particularly rocky time—at home, at school, or in the hospital setting. That's why it's important that therapy—whether group, individual, or simply a support network—continue over the long run. I will be discussing each of these different types of therapies, as well as others, later.

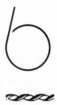

LEARNING DISABILITIES

It wasn't until fifteen months after Ronnie was born that his problems began. He crawled at eight months. He played "patty-cake" at nine months. He fed himself at eleven months. He asked to have his diaper changed at twelve months. He was chatty, healthy, and, if anything, a little shy with other playmates. But as Ronnie began his second year, he changed. Suddenly, he couldn't sit still. He couldn't focus his attention on anything more than a few moments at a time. He couldn't complete any projects, and he was impervious to discipline.

His parents were concerned, but they chalked up his behavior to being an energetic "little boy"—until he started school. His handwriting was poor; he had trouble retaining numbers and words. Soon he was behind all his other classmates, and he began to withdraw. By the time he finished third grade, his grades had dropped significantly. He was tested by a child evaluation team and was diagnosed as having learning disabilities: audio and visual memory impairment and poor fine motor skill control. Not being able to retain what he heard and saw meant Ronnie couldn't learn his ABC's or his multiplication tables. Not being able to coordinate his fingers meant he couldn't write well.

In the early part of the century, Alfred Binet joined forces with Theodore Simon to create a way to categorize children according to ability. They realized that a measure of intelligence had to be related to what a child could understand and discuss at a specific age—and they designed an intelligence test accordingly. But when Binet died, a man named Wilhelm Stern in Germany standardized Simon and Binet's concepts. He took a child's score (his mental age) and divided it by the average score of the entire group (the chronological age). This became the basis of our "I.Q."

But there was a crucial factor left out in Binet and Simon's initial testing: The boys had consistently lower scores than the girls. In fact, an average score for an entire group is invalid because boys develop more slowly than girls.

All three pioneers ignored this fact and changed the test so that any sex differences disappeared—and all intelligence tests since then have followed this practice. As Diane McGuinness points out in *When Children Don't Learn,* "All items that strongly favored girls were discarded and more items that favored boys were incorporated."

But Ronnie's I.Q. was also diagnosed as above normal. He was smart. He wanted to learn. When he couldn't, he became frustrated and scared. Learning became a horrendous chore. Instead of "knocking his head against the wall" by hopelessly trying to learn something in a way he was incapable of learning it, he grew frustrated—and literally knocked his head against the wall: he began acting out in class, talking out of turn, banging his desk, or simply staring off into space.

At home, he started yelling at his father. His mother, concerned and troubled, took Ronnie's side. She told her husband to have more patience. Soon Ronnie, an only child, was in the middle of a family feud—with no brothers or sisters to diffuse the flames.

Ronnie was sent to a special school in the seventh grade where, in his words, he was the "best student in his class." But the seeds of his learning disabilities had already taken root in the development of his self-esteem. Ronnie hated the fact that he was different, that he had to attend a special school. He had problems making friends and, though he had tried to get serious with a few girls he liked, he had no luck. In fact, a girl he'd started to date broke up with him just a week before I saw him for the first time.

Ronnie's parents brought him to Fair Oaks Hospital because he tried to kill himself with an overdose of his mother's Valium. Ronnie claimed he never wanted to commit suicide; he just wanted to "manipulate my parents and my girlfriend into helping me."

Ronnie was diagnosed as having a major depressive disorder. Though it was triggered by the stress of both his girlfriend's rejection and his family's fighting, Ronnie's depression was molded and augmented by his learning disabilities.

Ronnie had been put on medication for his hyperactivity and inattentiveness in the past—with little success. We decided to take a different tack. Instead of treating his inappropriate behavior, we treated both his depression and his problems with learning. Through individual, group, and family therapy, Ronnie learned to accept his learning disabilities. Special education programs and skill training helped him overcome his learning disabilities; he discovered different ways to learn. His self-esteem grew. And, the more peace he made with himself, the calmer he became.

By the time Ronnie was discharged, he was no longer depressed. His hyperactivity, his inattentiveness, his nervousness were all gone. He continued his therapy on an outpatient basis; his antidepressant medication was closely monitored. Today, he is in the tenth grade at his special school—and he is flourishing. The last time I saw him, he was making plans to study furniture design.

SYMPTOMS OF LEARNING DISABILITIES (LD)

- Has difficulty in keeping attention
- Shifts from one uncompleted activity to another
- Can't get organized or finish schoolwork
- Hands in messy homework
- Talks too much in class
- Is accident-prone
- Is noisy
- Is ready to do something dangerous without thinking of the consequences
- Initiates self-destructive activities on the spur of the moment
- Becomes a classic underachiever at school

These symptoms are only generalizations. Each one can signal either a variety of learning disabilities and hyperactivity or simply an individual teen's natural and normal development.

They will reflect LD if a child is born with cognitive vulnerabilities—which prevent him from processing his world as easily as do normal children. These vulnerabilities interact with the environment and produce learning disabilities. Although LD is present from the moment a child begins to explore and internalize his responses to his world, its symptoms usually coincide with starting school. For example, a child with impaired sensorimotor development will find he has trouble learning to write. He will grow frustrated and upset and begin to "act out" by handing in messy homework, by shifting from one uncompleted activity to another, or by displaying any of the other above symptoms.

The Unique Characteristics of LD

If we lived in a world of *Star Trek*'s Klingons, we'd admire aggression and force. If we lived in ancient Sparta, athletic prowess would win awards. If we lived in certain primitive tribes, our ability to grow food in abundance would make our mark. But we don't. Although our society applauds social charisma and athletic ability, math, reading, and spelling are needed to get ahead. According to Diane McGuinness, author of the excellent book *When Children Don't Learn,* the true definition of a learning disability is "the failure to learn anything at a normal rate, for whatever reason."

However, we don't call a teen "disabled" if he can't make a chocolate layer cake from a recipe—no matter how hard he tries. But if that same teen has trouble with reading or writing, the words "learning disabled" will soon appear on his school records. Why? Because in the same way other cultures give physical strength or a "green thumb" importance, we value reading, writing, and math above all.

Between 10 percent and 16 percent of all teenagers are called "learning disabled"—and that number soars up to 28 percent in urban school districts. But generalizations are dangerous, especially when they apply to LD. Many of these adolescents do indeed have learning problems— but many of them don't. It all comes down to a different set of "3 R's":

1. The Way Our Educational System Responds

Learning to tie your shoelaces is a skill routinely mastered anywhere from ages two to four. Learning to use a knife and fork also becomes routine during the toddler years. Learning to read and count is also a skill—but it is not mastered as commonly. Unfortunately, our traditional educational system gives literacy in language and math the same status as tied shoes and table manners by imposing deadlines for competency. By second grade, a child has to know his verbs. By third grade, he has to know how to construct a sentence. Often what looks like a learning disability is simply a slower rate of development—one that is perfectly normal for that particular teen.

The system simply doesn't take into account these natural differences between children. And, as Diane McGuinness also points out in her book: "Rather than fix the system, it is easier to blame the child."

2. The Relationship Between Boys and Girls

Boys and girls are different, and their minds and their bodies develop in different ways. Boys like to explore their world firsthand. This early "hands-on" approach gives boys the advantage in conceptualizing spatial relationships—and gives them the edge in higher mathematics. Girls are more verbal; they use language to learn. They gain the advantage in literacy because both their right and left brain hemispheres are involved in language—and they maintain a literacy lead of approximately two years during the developmental years.

But achievement tests don't take these biological and developmental differences into account. Even though girls are usually two years ahead of boys in verbal skills, achievement test scores use the combined average test scores of both sexes to determine who needs remedial help and who doesn't. This means that boys are being compared to girls who are two years ahead of them—with the result that 10 percent of all boys singled out for remedial reading are actually normal readers for their age and sex.

3. The Reasons for Learning Disabilities

Why can't Johnny read? Maybe because his parents are getting divorced, and there is so much strife in the family that he can't concentrate. Maybe it's the way he was raised—in a household where he was ignored or there was little emphasis put on education. Or maybe his teacher simply doesn't inspire a thirst for knowledge. None of these reasons involve actual learning disabilities. Yet more than one child has been mistakenly categorized as "disabled" because of them.

Approximately 2 to 8 percent of all school-age children develop a reading disorder, but it can be reversed with proper therapy and training. In fact, if your child has a reading disorder, he or she is in good company. Many successful people from all walks of life have had the same problem when they were young—including Thomas Edison, Woodrow Wilson, and Albert Einstein!

But if the reason Johnny couldn't read was because of perception impairment or memory dysfunction, he would be accurately diagnosed as having LD. Learning disabilities *always* involve a cognitive dysfunction in processing information—or, in other words, learning. Here, very briefly, are a few of the more common learning disorders.

DYSLEXIA. This is a general term used for many different kinds of reading disorders. Officially, dyslexia is a "developmental reading disorder." Children suffering from dyslexia usually have high I.Q.'s that contrast directly with their poor school performance. Dyslexics are usually boys who will distort, substitute, or omit words. They will also show signs of poor reading comprehension and they might read out loud in a slow, halting manner.

MATH BLOCKS. By the time a child is eight years old, a teacher can see that she has an inability to recognize math symbols or comprehend what numbers mean. She will have trouble memorizing multiplication and division tables, copying down equations, or counting. There are many developmental reasons why more girls have math blocks than boys, but sometimes society generates "math phobias." Even in today's more sophisticated times, the erroneous belief that "girls aren't good with math" is still considered fact by both males and females.

WRITING DISORDERS. Some teens can't write. They have trouble composing sentences or writing their thoughts down on paper. The essays they hand in will usually have spelling, punctuation, and organization mistakes. Most writing disorders are discovered by the time a child first starts to learn penmanship, but sometimes less severe cases aren't seen until a child is ten or older.

LANGUAGE DISORDERS. Because language becomes more and more complex with age, many teens who suffer from this disorder aren't diagnosed until they reach puberty. They will have a limited vocabulary and have difficulty learning new words. When they speak, they will use short sentences and, in some cases, unusual word orders. The prognosis for language disorders is good: between 3 percent and 10 percent of these teens are cured by the time they reach late adolescence.

SPEECH IMPEDIMENTS. Stuttering is the most obvious of all the speech problems—and its victims are three times more likely to be boys. "Speech on demand" will cause stuttering to accelerate, but when stutterers talk to their pets, sing, or engage in an easy conversation, their stuttering is almost nonexistent. Ninety-eight percent of all cases begin before a child is ten years old, but the condition takes several months to become a true impediment. Eighty percent of all stutters recover before they are sixteen—and 60 percent of that number without any benefit of speech therapy. Lisps and difficulties in pronouncing the *r, th, sh, f, z, ch,* or *l* sounds are as common as stuttering, and they too have a good cure rate with speech therapy.

There are many different types of learning disabilities within these broad categories. Your child can suffer from one of them—or from a combination of disorders at the same time. For example, if your child has dyslexia, she could also develop an expressive language disorder when she tries to read out loud or recite what she learned in class. Her symptoms can also vary from mild to very severe.

To understand exactly why these learning disabilities crop up the way they do, you must also understand the actual learning process— and the best way to do that is with a *cybernetic model.*

No, a cybernetic model is not a new robot for the latest *Star Wars* movie. Nor is it the latest toy to buy your child at Christmas. A cybernetic model, as used by scientists, explores the "drama" of human function. Here, it uses four components to explain how learning works—and how it can malfunction:

- *Input.* This is the process in which the brain receives information—via our perceptions from the five senses. A child sees his teacher point to the word "apple." He hears her say the word. If his perceptions are working correctly, he will understand what "apple" sounds like and how it is spelled—and send this new information to his brain. But if his auditory perception is impaired, he won't hear "apple." If he has dyslexia, he might transpose the "p" and the "a" and send faulty information to the brain for processing.
- *Integration.* Once the brain receives information, it must "settle in" with other pieces of information already there. A child without any disabilities will immediately associate the word "apple" with the real-life crunchy, juicy fruit that grows on trees. But a child suffering from a dysfunction of integration might not be able to make that word-picture connection. To him, "apples" might literally be "oranges."
- *Memory.* Now that the information is no longer new, it must be stored, to be retrieved at a moment's notice. The next time a

normal child sees the word "apple," he will remember it. He will not only associate "apple" with the crunchy, nutritious fruit—but with the one he ate yesterday afternoon while watching TV. A child with memory disabilities, however, will have trouble recalling the word "apple"—or remembering its connection to yesterday's snack.

- *Output.* The teacher is nodding to the normal child. She wants him to spell the word she had taught him. The child, perhaps a little nervous, perhaps a little unsure, stands up. His brain retrieves the word "apple" from his memory and sends it out to the world via speech. "A-p-p-l-e, apple," he says, relieved, conjuring up the visual word, the sound, the concept, and even the taste through language before he sits back down. But a child with an expressive language disability might stutter as he says "apple," especially when he is commanded to speak. He might have trouble visualizing the word in his mind. Confused, he spells it wrong.

A learning disability can only occur when there is a malfunction in this learning process. But some children are more susceptible to this condition than others. There are three influences that come into play:

1. "It really hurt when this girl I liked started to giggle when I couldn't read that section from *Julius Caesar*"

Seventy-five percent of all dyslexics are boys. Some studies suggest this is due to sexual hormonal growth; the male hormone testosterone has been found to delay left hemisphere growth in the brain. Because of this delayed growth, boys have verbal capabilities in only one hemisphere. Thus, they are predisposed to language disorders if their early cognitive development has left them vulnerable.

But girls also have disorders—especially when it comes to math. While girls are busy learning through language, boys, as we have seen, are learning with their hands—developing at an early age an aptitude for visualizing objects in space. This understanding of spatial relationships helps them when it comes to geometry, algebra, and calculus. Conversely, a girl's lack of interest in hands-on exploration creates problems in spatial relationships and possible math phobias. In fact, a study by the Johns Hopkins University of both boys' and girls' Scholastic Aptitude Test scores found that *only boys* had exceptionally high scores in the advanced math sections.

2. "My dad has no interest in reading, and I guess I don't, either"

Learning disabilities run in families. A seven-year study of more than 29,000 children found that the strongest predictor of a child developing LD was the fact that his siblings had a learning disorder, too. Other studies have found that children are more at risk for developing the same LD their parents had—if one or both were learning disabled. Adopted children are also not immune. If their natural parents were learning disabled, the chances are greater that they will be, too.

But environment also plays a role. That same seven-year study of 29,000 children also found that learning disabilities were more prevalent in families that moved frequently, had many family members, or were in a poorer socioeconomic class.

Learning takes time and patience. Parents under stress might not be able to give a child the attention he needs—especially if they have to give equal time to many different siblings. Consequently, this child's cognitive development can be stymied and result in a learning disability.

3. "I hate school. I'll always hate school"

The school environment functions as a detective; it is the place where learning disabilities are usually discovered—in the first few grades. Here a child first begins to do reading, writing, and arithmetic in earnest, and a teacher can see if he isn't reading up to par, if he's transposing letters when he spells, if he can't write his name.

It is also around school age that some children will develop the psychological symptoms of LD. By the time a child is seven years old, he has learned some social skills; he has a sense of who he is and what his responsibilities are. But a learning disabled child is continually frustrated. He can't learn. This frustration leads to boredom—which can often lead to depression, inattentiveness, and aggressive acting out. Worse, he begins to associate learning with pain. If he isn't helped, he will stop wanting to learn—and he won't try as hard. A study of both healthy and handicapped toddlers discovered that the handicapped children didn't work as hard to complete a task because they simply didn't believe they'd succeed. This study also indicates that a "loser" mentality emerges at a very early age. Over time, it only grows, along with its accompanying low self-esteem, depression, and anger.

To show this insidious pattern at work, let's jump ten years into the future and visit a learning disabled student in his English class. He sits in the back of the room, head against the bulletin board, eyes closed. His copy of *A Tale of Two Cities* is upside down; he has drawn all over the pages. He begins to snore in a loud, intentional manner. All he wants is for the bell to ring.

This teenager stopped trying to do well in school a long time ago. He does anything he can to get out of it. His teachers complain because he constantly makes jokes and talks out of turn. His parents complain because his grades are bad. He won't admit it to himself, but he's embarrassed. He feels guilty that he's let everybody down. To keep these feelings at bay, he acts out even more. Maybe he breaks the cafeteria window. Maybe he starts hanging out with those other guys who don't bother to go to school. Maybe he starts doing drugs to ease the pain. Maybe these are the only ways he can feel like something—or someone.

This scenario is simplistic, but the facts are clear: A learning disability can lead to frustration and failure, which in turn lead to poor self-esteem. This poor self-image soon permeates every area of a learning disabled teen's life and creates a trap of depression, withdrawal, or aggressive and antisocial behavior. It's no wonder that a learning disability is the number-one reason why teenagers drop out of school. LD can be a vicious catalyst, and I'll be discussing its power at length in the next chapter on conduct disorders.

Learning disabilities are often at the root of inappropriate behavior. But this fact is often forgotten in the onslaught of a teenager's dramatic acting out. Instead of looking beneath the surface, parents often mistake a learning disability for the inappropriate behavior itself. Overactivity, aggression, inattention—all might be symptoms of a learning disorder and not an attention-deficit hyperactivity disorder.

ATTENTION-DEFICIT HYPERACTIVITY DISORDER (ADHD)

Craig is six years old and, though it hasn't yet been diagnosed, he has a memory retention disability and an audio perception problem. He is wandering around upstairs and enters his mother's room. She's cleaning and realizes that she left her dust mop downstairs. When she sees Craig, she asks him to get it for her. Craig, grinning, says, "Sure, Mommy!" He enthusiastically bounds down the stairs—but he suddenly stops. He forgot what she wanted. He has to go back upstairs and ask his mother again. She wants to finish her housework; she's annoyed that Craig didn't get the mop. "See, you don't listen to me. Why can't you do what I ask?" Craig is crestfallen. He agrees with his mom; he's a bad boy. He can't yet verbalize—or understand—his problem.

The scene shifts. Craig is in school. His teacher usually writes the homework assignment on the blackboard. But the bell has just rung for recess and she doesn't have time. Instead, she explains the assignment out loud. Craig listens and tries to understand—but it's a little fuzzy. He doesn't know that he has a memory retention problem when he hears—but doesn't see—something. He doesn't realize that if his teacher had written the assignment down, he would have read it, understood it, and remembered it. Craig is only six. He simply doesn't have the ability to realize that he can only remember things that are written down. Instead, he continues to forget what he is told.

It's a year later. Craig has become a frustrated student. He's bored, he's turned off—and he's easily distracted. After all, he's tried to listen to the teacher and it just doesn't make any sense. So why pay attention? He'd much rather run around the room. Or bang his head on the desk. Or talk really, really loud. Unfortunately, like every child, Craig must sit in a classroom and learn.

Most studies of children with ADHD dwell on the hyperactive symptoms—and whether or not drug therapy works. But one recent study of fifty-seven children was different. Here, Major Peter S. Jensen, M.D., Lieutenant Colonel Michael W. Bain, M.D., and Dr. Allen M. Josephson attempted to discover the psychological effects of the drugs given ADHD children. They found that the drugs were successful in treating the ADHD symptoms, but taking a pill several times a day left psychological scars, including a loss of self-esteem, an ingrained belief that the child has to take a "good pill" because he's a "bad boy," and, because the child seems "cured," a continuation of the underlying family stress and problems that might have triggered the ADHD.

Here are some of the questions the interviewers asked the children:

"What's the name of the pill you take?"

"What does the pill do?"

"What is wrong with you that you have to take a pill?"

"Were you always hyper?"

. . . And some of their replies:

"Maybe something damaged my brain at birth, because now I am like the Incredible Hulk, because if I get mad, I get red in the face, can't control myself, and might even hit my best friend in the face!"

"No, I haven't always been hyper, just after my mom and dad got divorced, and then we had to move here. I want to go back and live with my dad, but my mom won't let me."

Medication works, but it is not a "magic bullet." Parents must participate in family therapy. The pills must be monitored and a child must not be blamed for the tension his illness has caused. His self-esteem must be enhanced through patience, understanding, and support.

Within the next few weeks, Craig is diagnosed as having attention-deficit hyperactivity disorder (ADHD). He is given medication for his hyperactivity. He's calmed down a little—but he still isn't doing well in school. He still doesn't participate in class or join his peers in a game of kickball during recess. The impact of this situation on his life is enormous. Instead of treating the learning disability, teaching him new ways to learn to help him cope and build up his self-esteem, he is being treated for hyperactivity—which in this case is only a symptom of the underlying LD. It's not the disorder itself. Craig is calm—but he's far from well.

Ten years ago, it was called hyperactivity. Today, the phrase is ADHD—but it's still the same disorder. Over 200,000 elementary school children are estimated to have ADHD—and 90 percent of them are boys. The symptoms are very much like those of learning disabilities, but with these crucial differences:

1. ADHD: Overall problems in learning.
   LD: A *specific* dysfunction within the learning process.
2. ADHD: Hyperactivity a result of a chemical imbalance in the brain.
   LD: Hyperactivity only a symptom of the learning disorder.
3. ADHD: Infants usually exhibit irritable behavior. They don't play in one activity for too long. They sleep very little. They wear out clothes, toys—and a mother's patience—very fast.
   LD: Infants can develop normally. The learning disorder doesn't always show up until the child is in school.
4. ADHD: Children are very uncoordinated and very fidgety in class.
   LD: Children are usually less fidgety. Can be better in sports.
5. ADHD: There is a strong genetic link. Studies have found that if both fathers and uncles have had ADHD when they were younger, the chances are great that their sons and nephews will develop it, too.
   LD: Can also be inherited. But it is the basic disorder that is passed on—not the hyperactive symptoms.
6. ADHD: Symptoms are seen in *all* situations.
   LD: Symptoms are usually confined to the situations where the disability might crop up. For example, an LD teen might sit and daydream during English, but he will enthusiastically participate in shop.
7. ADHD: There is a prompt positive response to medication.
   LD: Medication will calm children down—but only to a certain extent. They will continue to have problems in a school environment.

I hope that this list will help you wade through the mistaken identity "plot" that occurs whenever LD or ADHD appears—because I am about to add a bit more. Just as a learning disability can be mistaken for ADHD, an attention-deficit disorder itself is sometimes misdiagnosed.

People are quick to blame ADHD when they see a child acting "hyper." But a child can have ADHD without racing through the aisles. The emphasis of ADHD falls on the first two words: "attention deficit." The disorder literally means a lack of attention—which has nothing to do with a child's level of activity. Inattention can mean gazing out the window just as much as it means running around a room. attention-deficit disorders can develop with—or without—hyperactive symptoms.

In fact, hyperactivity without a sustained loss of attention can actually be normal behavior and not signal ADHD or an underlying learning disability at all. Both children and teens relieve anxiety by increasing their muscle activity. Jangling legs, bouncing pencils, tapping fingers on desk "drums"—all can just be nerves.

Depression can also cause overactivity. When parents are inconsistent or overbearing, their children can become confused, anxious, and erratic, and look, to all the world, as if they have ADHD or learning problems.

Learning disabilities. Attention-deficit disorders. Hyperactivity. All are related. All can be combined. Unfortunately, between 60 percent and 80 percent of ADHD children become teens who have problems with school performance, self-image, their relationships with their peers, distinguishing right from wrong, and taking responsibility for their actions. They can become delinquents suffering from conduct disorders. A longitudinal study of hyperactive children who are now adults found that half of them outgrew their behavior. Unfortunately, the half that didn't outgrow their hyperactivity grew up with low-self esteem, broken relationships, and a predisposition toward antisocial behavior. As this study proves, a correct diagnosis in childhood is crucial. The proper help can prevent a negative self-fulfilling prophecy from coming true as your teen struggles to adulthood.

Treating Learning Disabilities
Treating the learning disability instead of the ADHD symptoms can result in better behavior. Giving a teen the skills he needs to learn and build up his self-esteem will stop those feelings of rejection, frustration, and self-loathing that cause him to act out.

At hospitals like Fair Oaks we try to teach our learning-disabled teens new approaches and new tools for learning. It's important for these teens to put their problem into perspective. Even people without LD have learned to learn better. Some people prefer bringing a tape recorder to a lecture. Others like to take notes. Still others like to underline. The methods don't matter as long as the information can be learned.

DIET AND ADHD

In 1982 when allergist Dr. Benjamin Feingold proposed that hyperactivity could be controlled by eliminating food additives and artificial colorings, his "Feingold Diet" became an immediate hit among parents of ADHD children. But subsequent studies have not been able to prove that the diet controls any hyperactivity. Children have been known to calm down with the Feingold Diet, but this may be due to the fact that, in order to stick with the program, they are receiving a great deal of attention and focus from their parents.

Part of the difficulty in treating LD is making an accurate diagnosis in the first place. Many teens with learning problems are fine in one-on-one situations. Dyslexics, for example, have been known to read just fine when they've picked out a book for some "private time." And children with ADHD have sat quietly talking to a therapist for hours.

Further, a learning disability does not always show up during neurological tests. "Minimal brain damage" means nothing in most cases. Children with slight brain damage can learn without any problems. And children with normal brain function can have LD. Both minimal brain damage and neurological soft signs have been bandied about by people as much as the term "hyperactivity." But, in most cases, they signify nothing.

A learning disability, however, can be pinpointed through extensive psychological testing—including a patient's documented lifeline and a thorough physical exam.

If a child is diagnosed as having ADHD, medications such as Ritalin and Dexedrine have been proven to help a great deal. The main reason there is so much controversy over these drugs is that the ADHD might have been misdiagnosed in the first place—or that an underlying learning disability is being ignored. I will be discussing these medications as well as many others in chapter eleven.

The good news is that many learning disorders disappear by the time your child reaches puberty. But if your child has become a teenager and is still suffering from the pain of LD, there is hope. Learning disabilities can be dealt with in alternative education programs, remedial reading, tutoring, and speech therapy. The depression a learning disability causes can be treated with medication in combination with individual, group, and family therapy.

I remember a boy who had been diagnosed as having dyslexia. When he first came to Fair Oaks Hospital's Adolescent Unit, he read nothing more than the results of the latest Mets game. Today, seven years later, he is preparing his thesis on moral responsibility in *Crime and Punishment.*

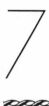

CONDUCT DISORDERS

His history sounded like a cliché: an alcoholic mother, a brother who was a drug addict, and a father who had walked out over six years ago. When he was seven, he tried to stop his father from hitting his mother. When he was eight, he watched his mother try to kill herself. When he was twelve, he helped his brother forge one of his stepfather's checks. When he was fifteen, he was suspended from school for carrying a knife.

His name was Sam and he'd undeniably experienced a lot for a sixteen-year-old boy. I saw him a few months after he'd been suspended. He'd had a number of violent outbursts at home: screaming at his stepfather, breaking a lamp and a coffee table, and, two days prior to his admission to Fair Oaks, threatening his mother with a knife. "I feel like everyone is out to get me—even the people who are trying to calm me down," he told me the afternoon I met him in my office. "I've become like a wild animal."

But Sam wasn't always this way. He made the honor roll five times in elementary school. His development appeared normal. He'd even helped his mother around the house when he was small, drying dishes, dusting, and feeding his goldfish. He and his mother were very close; he'd always run to her when she and his father fought. Unfortunately, this would make his father even angrier; he would look at Sam with disgust.

The problems began when his mother started drinking. Suddenly, Sam didn't have his "security." The trauma of his mother's suicide attempt stayed with him. He poured the water out of his fishbowl and watched his goldfish die. He drew vivid murals on his bedroom walls. He began wetting his bed. He started sleeping in his mother's room, a habit he continued until he was fourteen years old.

When his father left the house, the family atmosphere improved—until Sam's brother began taking drugs. Sam's bed-wetting started up again, and his brother taunted him, calling him a baby. Even his mother seemed annoyed; she told him it was "time you grew up." Sam was confused. Maybe he was a baby; maybe he needed his mother too much. There was only one thing to do: avoid his feelings at all costs.

Sam soon learned that screaming had an effect—especially when he broke things or wielded a knife. It was called power. Instead of feeling humiliated, he could humiliate others. By controlling others, he kept their ability to control him at bay.

By the time Sam started junior high school, his aggressiveness was intact. Teachers, parents, peers: no one was going to tell him what to do. His grades started falling. His mother, who had started biweekly therapy sessions, insisted that Sam see a therapist. He went for several months, then abruptly quit.

Things went from bad to worse. Sam started hanging out with older boys and cutting school. His mother attempted to set up some rules. The first night she gave him a curfew, he ran away for twenty-four hours. The day he was caught writing graffiti on a neighborhood store, she paid his fine and grounded him for a week. He ran away again.

Soon Sam became uncontrollable. His stepfather "washed his hands of him." His mother looked at him with hurt and helpless eyes. Only violent outbursts helped.

"I would like to take back every time that I blew up," Sam said when he'd been at Fair Oaks Hospital for a month. At Fair Oaks, Sam was put on medication to help control his wild mood swings. Family therapy helped change the atmosphere at home and make discipline, routine, and responsibility more consistent. Individual therapy helped him understand the dynamics of disappointment and fear underlying his behavior. Behavioral therapy helped him develop better moral and social skills. And the hospital setting itself set up boundaries and rules to help him learn to control his impulses. Sam will be discharged in another month. He will be going back to his neighborhood high school.

He will live at home and continue his therapy on an outpatient basis.

Now ready to go back to his life, Sam has accepted the fact that his family will never be "perfect," that he will never get the kind of love and security he wants from them. He has also learned the new power of communication, which he can use to talk out his anger and frustration—instead of acting out. Sam is ready to grow up, and the prognosis looks good.

The Symptoms of Conduct Disorders

Three or more of these symptoms lasting for at least six months could signal a conduct disorder—and the need for intervention:

- Stealing, without confronting a victim, more than once (including forgery)
- Running away overnight at least twice (or once without returning home)
- Lying often
- Engaging in deliberate fire-setting
- Cutting school often
- Breaking into someone else's house, building, or car
- Deliberately destroying someone's property
- Physical cruelty to animals
- Forcing sexual activity on others
- Using a weapon in more than one fight
- Stealing by confronting a victim, including mugging, purse-snatching, extortion, and armed robbery
- Physically abusing people

These symptoms can be mild, when only minor harm has been suffered by others, or severe, when considerable pain has been inflicted—such as serious physical injury, extensive vandalism, and prolonged absences from home.

Symptoms are one thing. The way a conduct-disordered teen behaves is another. There are three distinct behavioral patterns and three distinct "players":

THE LONER. The **DSM-III-R** categorizes this type of conduct disorder as *solitary aggressive.* This teen will make little attempt to cover up his antisocial behavior. Indeed, he might even boast about his exploits. He is undersocialized, which means what it says: He is socially isolated and unable to get along with his parents or his peers.

THE GANG MEMBER. The **DSM-III-R** calls this a *group type*. This teen works in groups, sometimes as a physically aggressive "team player" and sometimes as a passive follower. Because he will commit his antisocial acts only with the other members of his gang, he is also considered by the DSM-III-R as *socialized nonaggressive*. His friends, his self-esteem, his loyalty—all are powerfully tied to the gang.

THE BLACK SHEEP. This teen is the exception to the rule. A conduct-disordered teen can give his loyalty to a group that doesn't want him. He can be a sneaky and devious loner, committing his antisocial activities in a "passive-aggressive" way to get what he wants. Because conduct-disordered adolescents can be both socialized and aggressive, undersocialized and nonaggressive, or any other combination of the two, the DSM-III-R calls this the *undifferentiated type*.

In a landmark study of fifty-five juvenile delinquents, Drs. Daniel Offer, R. C. Marohn, and Eric Ostrov discovered four distinct types of conduct-disordered teens:

- **The Impulsive**—has little self-control. He needs immediate gratification and is unable to make plans or goals constructively. He is ready for anything—which usually means violent antisocial acts.
- **The Narcissistic**—can only preserve his self-esteem by acting out. He takes grandiose poses and uses other people to temporarily fill in the empty places of his soul. He views himself as completely well-adjusted, but others see him as manipulative and superficial.
- **The Depressed Borderline**—is actually well-liked. He takes the initiative in school, but feels a great deal of depression and guilt. He "acts out" as a way to relieve this inner pain.
- **The Empty Borderline**—is very passive, unpopular, and emotionally bereft. To reduce his empty, hopeless, and sometimes psychotic thoughts, he will act out in deviant, aggressive ways.

The Unique Characteristics of Conduct Disorders

We all know the scenario. The boy from the wrong side of the tracks, the leather jacket, the guns, the gangs, the rage. But underneath this James Dean demeanor is a troubled teen in pain, a child who has stopped asking for love because he believes there is no hope.

Unfortunately, this lack of hope is often a reality. Conduct-disordered teens are hard to take. They can be cruel, violent, and dangerous. It's difficult for them to gain our sympathy—or motivate us to offer help. In fact, CD is considered the one disorder that inflicts more pain on others than within its victim.

But if your child is suffering from a conduct disorder, you know you need to reach him or her—and it is possible. But you must understand what—and who—you are dealing with. Like a complex role in a serious play, the conduct-disordered personality contains many underlying characteristics. Let's go over them now.

THE ADHD CONNECTION. It's true. A child suffering from attention-deficit hyperactive disorder can develop into a conduct-disordered teen. In fact, a longitudinal study of 101 teenage boys who had been diagnosed as hyperactive as children found that the greatest risk factor for developing conduct disorders was the persistence of ADHD symptoms. Other research bears this out: A study of 110 adolescent boys with ADHD and 88 normal boys found that there was a higher rate of delinquency among the ADHD subjects. Another study found that among children diagnosed as hyperactive, 43 percent continued to have emotional, learning, and behavioral problems in their teens.

The key word here is "persistent." Children who no longer have ADHD symptoms when they reach adolescence are at no more risk than normal children for developing a conduct disorder. But if the impulsiveness, the inattention, and the hyperactivity continue through the teenage years, the risk increases. The hyperactivity ADHD children show by running around a room becomes the fuel to break windows or steal when they become teenagers. Their impulsiveness becomes more and more a lack of responsible, good judgment. Their poor social development becomes the catalyst for deviant, amoral, and antisocial behavior.

Although a persistent ADHD is considered a predictor of CD, it is this antisocial behavior that separates the two. As we have seen in chapter six, the main symptom of attention-deficit disorder is inattention—which does not automatically translate into antisocial acts. A careful diagnosis must be made by a mental health professional before a teen is labeled a juvenile delinquent.

THE LEARNING DISABILITY PROLOGUE. Like ADHD, many conduct disorders have a learning disability at their root—especially reading and language disorders. A teen who can't read or understand words cannot verbalize his feelings or his thoughts. His only mode of communication is action. And, because of his frustration and its accompanying low self-esteem, this action is usually angry and antisocial.

How can you tell if a learning disability is the culprit? A study by Dr. Michael Rutter found that teenagers who developed conduct disorders between the ages of ten and fourteen had no higher a percentage of learning disorders than the general population. But teenagers who developed conduct disorders before the age of ten were almost always saddled with a learning disability as well.

THE HOUSE THAT CD BUILT. Deviant parents make deviant children. A study by Drs. Eleanor Glueck and Sheldon Glueck found that 84 percent of delinquents in Massachusetts reformatories already had criminals within their family.

This makes sense. As we have seen earlier, parents are a child's first role model for socialization. If they are aggressive and antisocial, their children will imitate them—and learn to be antisocial as well. Siblings will also imitate each other. Studies have found that they too can become delinquent if one of their brothers or sisters already is.

Sometimes it's not the overt antisocial behavior that creates CD. A child can also take on the repressed antisocial drives that his parents would never address. Called superego lacunae by Drs. A.M. Johnson and Stanislaus Szurek, this condition motivates children not only to commit their deviant acts—but to commit them without any guilt.

However, parents do not have to be antisocial themselves. A couple's alcoholism, abuse, depression, or inadequate development can all be conveyed to their child—creating stress that, in the absence of someone to teach adequate coping skills, finds an outlet in antisocial acts and aggression. Studies bear this out: Mothers of delinquent children have been found to be inconsistent, tense, frustrated, and less mature. Fathers of delinquent children have been found to be inadequate and emotionally distant. The good news is that one supportive parent can counteract the negative child-rearing practices of the other and reduce the risk of their child developing a conduct disorder. But there's more to a conduct disorder than this "parent trap." There are several other factors that make up the dysfunctional family and its resulting CD.

1. The Communication Factor

Families with conduct-disordered teens have poor and defensive lines of communication. Messages of aggressive power and control, statements that are judgmental and absolute, words that convey angry indifference to other people and conversations that only attempt to impress others are all defensive ways of communicating—which leads to defensive "acting out." Problems never get discussed or solved. And sensitivity to a troubled teen never surfaces in any room of the house.

2. The Discipline Factor

Discipline with love might sound like a cliché, but parents who practice consistent discipline with less physical punishment and more patient reasoning have children who develop healthy self-control. On the other hand, parents who practice severe and inconsistent physical punishment raise children who have little self-control and who, more times than not, develop conduct disorders.

Lying is a symptom of both conduct disorders and oppositional defiant disorders. But, as we all know, there are different degrees of lying—from white lies to aggressive, cruel lies. Children themselves can go through three processes of lying:

1. "The Incredible Hulk came to the house today."
   When very young children lie it is more like wishful thinking. Their lies are as innocent as they themselves are; they believe what they say.
2. "My parents are taking me to Disney World next week."
   As children develop and grow, they learn frustration. They tell fantasy lies. They wish what they were saying was true, but they know it isn't.
3. "Mrs. Rose asked me to be a cheerleader yesterday without even a tryout. But I had to tell her no. I'm just too busy."

If a child has reached her teens and is still telling lies, it is a sign of impaired moral development and she is considered a "delinquent liar." She might lie to gain a material object, to protect herself from a fearful authority figure, to escape criticism or punishment, or, as in the above example, to appear better than she feels she is. In fact, a study found that teens who cheat in school usually do so because they are trapped between "a rock and a hard place." The rock is high parental expectation. The hard place is limited abilities that prevent success.

In fact, the consistency of discipline is more important than whether it is severe or overly lax. But inconsistency is more than a sometime punishment. If an authoritative, hostile father metes out the punishment while an indifferent, permissive mother stands by, inconsistency rears its head and creates aggression in the confused teen. If a father, because of his own impaired development, inappropriately responds positively to his son's aggression, this too creates inconsistency. Here's an example: John's school suspended him for cutting classes three days in a row. His father was furious—and hit him when he came home. Then when John hit a neighborhood boy who had teased him about the suspension, his father was pleased. "No one calls my son a bum." If John had tried to use reason with the neighborhood boy instead of hitting him, his father would have called him a "sissy." John's father used inconsistent discipline—which only reinforced John's antisocial behavior.

Reinforcement also comes from lack of interest. Studies have found that, on the whole, parents of conduct-disordered teens are more distant and unfriendly. They won't believe it when they hear that their child has stolen a bike out of the schoolyard or a carton of soda from the neighborhood store. They won't confront their son unless they have substantial evidence—not out of pain or fear, but out of disinterest for their roles as parent-teachers, for the values of society, and for their child himself. This only reinforces their son's bad behavior. Dr. G.R. Patterson calls this a "coercive family process" in which the child's deviant behavior is supported or reinforced by the parent—which in turn continues to reinforce the behavior in the child. Further, this confusing reinforcement can also be a reason why CD teens are less responsive to rewards and punishments than normal children.

3. The Disorganized Factor

Erratic discipline, moody parents, and erratic household routines and rules make for inconsistency—and can lead to CD. When it comes to organization, large families can have a difficult time. There is less interaction between parents and children and more between siblings, which can also give rise to a conduct disorder.

4. The Single Parent Factor

Studies show that many conduct-disordered teens come from homes disrupted by desertion, divorce, and death. Other studies show that most incarcerated teens suffer from parental separation and loss.

Earlier, we saw that the family discord that precedes a separation is more harmful to a developing child than the actual divorce itself. In fact, a teen's antisocial behavior increases the more his parents' relationship deteriorates. Boys from homes where discord abounds have been found to be more impulsive, more antisocial, less self-controlled, less able to delay immediate gratification, and more rebellious against adult authority figures than boys whose home life is intact.

The actual divorce reduces the discord that creates these behaviors. But even though the arguments and the fighting have stopped, a single-parent household still has many unique conflicts and stresses that can create a conduct disorder in a teenager. Because mothers usually retain custody of their children, studies have focused on these single-mother homes. They have found that single mothers often:

- Are overburdened with responsibility and tasks.
- Are financially strapped.
- Feel trapped and take it out on their children—especially the teen who is already acting out.
- Discipline less effectively than fathers—who, studies have found, are listened to more seriously than mothers.
- Offer only one parental role model to emulate—with no buffer to separate the positive and negative elements
- Are socially isolated with no emotional and social support.

5. The Class Factor

Poverty, inadequate housing, and abuse—all are factors why conduct disorders are more prevalent in low socioeconomic classes. These poor conditions not only result in conduct disorders—but they can also make it worse. For example, physical abuse is often found in families where financial and marital support is lacking, where there is a history of abuse in the family, and where depression is rampant—situations that occur more frequently in lower-class families. A conduct-disordered child from this troubled lower-class family might be severely punished—but without consistency. This type of discipline, as we have seen, creates more antisocial behavior. But the physical abuse itself also has far-reaching implications. Severe abuse can result in brain damage, learning disability, ADHD, central nervous system dysfunction, and poor impulse control, all of which perpetuate the conduct disorder. In addition, the by-products of low socioeconomic classes—poor housing, malnutrition, neglect, and lead poisoning, among others—have all been found to lead to additional aggressiveness in troubled teens.

6. The City Factor

The city can truly be a "rat race." Conduct disorder is found much more frequently in teenagers living in metropolitan areas than in the country. Why? Rural crimes are rarely committed against other people; minor vandalism and "driving under the influence" are more the norm. In a survey of rural Ohio residents, teenage vandalism, especially damage to mailboxes, was the number-one complaint. Larceny came in second. Another difference: The types of teenage crime that occur in the country would not receive police attention in the city. A study of 187 rural jails and detention centers found that 55 percent of the youthful offenders would have been ineligible for incarceration in metropolitan areas.

The fact is that city life can be dangerous. Conduct-disorder rates are much lower in rural areas—as are rates for other emotional disturbances in children, teenagers, and adults.

ONE-MAN SHOW. It was always this way: Billy would curse at a teacher—and blame her for provoking him. He would get into a fistfight at school, because the other kid always started it first. He would steal the family car for a joyride—and tell his parents he wouldn't take it again if they'd let him have his own set of wheels. After all, Billy is terrific; there's nothing wrong with him. It's his teachers, his parents, or the other kids at school who are the problem. Whenever Billy commits a deviant act, it's because of something someone else did—or didn't do.

Billy displays a typical characteristic of a conduct disorder: egocentricity. Quite simply, these teens believe the world revolves around them. They can do no wrong. Rather than taking responsibility for themselves, teens with conduct disorder blame the outside world. To admit otherwise would mean a loss of control—and, as Dr. Daniel Offer discovered in his study of juvenile delinquents, a lack of control is the most terrifying emotion a conduct-disordered teen can face. It is far less painful to point the finger of blame at someone else—and consider himself "hot" and "above it all." In fact, Dr. Offer also discovered that conduct-disordered teens have a surprisingly good self-image. They consider themselves physically attractive, strong, and hip. They have to be this egocentric—or they will crumble.

Think about it: A conduct-disordered teen has probably spent his younger years frustrated and confused over his learning disabilities, his ADHD, his family strife. He's developed patterns of lying and cheating. His poor impulse control has led him from desire to immediate action—without leaving room or time in between for judgment. His inability to express his confusion and feelings of inadequacy verbally has led to years of frustration. As this frustration grows, it seethes with power and explodes into violent hostility.

He's now a teenager saddled with this hostility. He's gone from setting fires and cutting school to armed robbery. He's started hanging out with other "JDs"; they bolster each other up. They might be considered outsiders, but they know they are the only game in town. The kids who achieve in school, who join the football team and go to dances are the "jerks." Real guys take dangerous risks. They experiment with drugs and develop substance abuse problems which, as studies prove, often follow the onset of a conduct disorder. They learn to feel a sense of control and mastery with every drag race, with every "hit."

But drugs, gangs, and violence are not a part of our real, constructive world. These teens are, as psychologist Erik Erikson said, "pseudocompetent." They are only faking it—and deep inside they know it. In fact, a study of sixty teenagers with conduct disorders discovered that eleven of them also classified as having a major depression. Underneath these CD teens' egocentricity and hostility lie feelings of worthlessness—without any outlet for their hostility but antisocial acts.

THE BIOLOGY REVUE. The body cannot be separated from the mind. In addition to the psychological reasons for conduct disorders, there are the reasons rooted in genetics and physiology. Studies of adopted children have found that if a natural father is a criminal, a child can grow up to be a criminal too—regardless of his adoptive home. If his adoptive father is also deviant, the risk is even higher.

The good news is that the total risk of inheriting a conduct disorder is much less than in other disorders. It is, rather, the dysfunctional family circle—with its alcoholism, antisocial behaviors, depression, and abuse—that contributes to CD. Other biological aspects of conduct disorders can be inherited. Autonomic nervous system arousal has been found to be deficient in people who commit antisocial acts. This translates into a decreased response to stimulation—which has implications for the socialization process. Here's how, according to Drs. S.A. Mednick and B. Hutchings:

1. A child contemplates an aggressive act.
2. He experiences fear induced by "remembrances of punishments past."
3. His impulse to commit the aggressive act is inhibited.
4. Consequently, his fear diminishes.

This dissipation of fear is the strongest psychological reinforcer for keeping aggression at bay. But teens with slow autonomic nervous system arousal cannot respond to the inhibiting stimulus of fear. Instead, they plunge in and commit their aggressive act.

Then there's the element of serotonin, a chemical neurotransmitter that relays messages throughout the brain. Serotonin's presence is crucial for our minds to work normally. When imbalances in serotonin levels occur, the results can be depression, anxiety, and conduct disorder. Its levels have been found to be lower in "loner" conduct-disorder types and higher in "gang member" oversocialized types. Brain wave abnormalities have also been found in conduct-disordered boys while they are asleep.

In his book *Castaways,* author George Cadwalader describes a scene he could have witnessed one moonlit night at his Outward Bound program for juvenile delinquents on Penikese Island off the New England coast. One of the teens broke into the compound's chicken coop. There, he systematically broke the legs of each and every chicken in the coop.

Cruelty to animals is a devastating symptom of a conduct disorder. It is not the one-time violent act that insures later violence toward people. Rather, it is the recurrent cruelty that accurately predicts later conduct disorders. A child who continuously tortures the family cat, the child who remains fascinated by dog, cock, or bull fights, the child who turns a deaf ear to an animal in pain—these are signs of early aggression that, as with the teen who broke the chickens' legs, will result in later delinquency and violence toward people.

Finally, there is the physiological component of temperament. As we have seen in chapter one, children are born with three different types of temperament: difficult, easy, and slow-to-warm-up. Children who develop conduct disorders grew up, more often than not, with a difficult temperament. Perhaps their parents reacted to their crankiness by unconsciously rejecting them. Perhaps they received more negative feedback. Perhaps their irritability made them more susceptible to developmental problems later on. Whatever the reason, in some cases, a difficult child's temperament can be prophetic and result in aggression.

BOYS AND GIRLS TOGETHER. Boys who develop conduct disorders outnumber girls three to one. Why? Some scientists say it's because high levels of testosterone are found in conduct-disordered teens. Others say it's a component of an abnormal Y chromosone configuration. Still others say it's because girls are more verbal than boys—and they are able to voice their pain more easily. And still others say it's because girls are taught to inhibit their aggression by both their parents and society at large. Instead of unruliness, the focus is on sexual behavior. Research bears this out: While boys act out their aggression in destructive, violent ways, girls with conduct disorders become sexually promiscuous.

There is also a pattern to conduct disorders. Deviant boys will start out slowly in early adolescence, breaking windows in empty houses, sneaking free rides on public transportation, and shoplifting from local stores. By seventeen their aggression will peak and aimless acts of vandalism will evolve into burglary, armed robbery, and dealing in stolen goods—all of which, more times than not, result in guilty verdicts. In fact, stealing is the number-one crime committed by conduct-disordered teens.

In a way, a conduct disorder is a rainstorm that has developed into a hurricane. The learning disability, the dysfunctional family, the ADHD, the underlying low self-esteem—all were there in childhood and, without help at that time, they've been blown out of proportion. Careening out of control, the anger swirls and the hostility builds—until relief is found in disruptive, antisocial behavior.

But there is another disorder that follows this same pattern, one that is often confused with CD. It's called *oppositional defiant disorder* (ODD) and its symptoms include:

- Losing their temper
- Arguing with adults
- Defying adults
- Deliberately doing something to annoy others
- Blaming others for their own mistakes
- Being touchy and easily annoyed
- Feeling angry and resentful
- Acting spiteful and vindictive
- Swearing often

If the ODD symptoms sound very similar to those of a conduct disorder, they should. Studies have found ODD to be more a mild form of CD than a separate illness. The main differences between the two are that:

1. More girls suffer from ODD than from conduct disorder.
2. Teens who have ODD do not violate the rights of others to the same degree as those with a conduct disorder.

But whether your teen is suffering from ODD or CD, treatment is always necessary. Let's go on to the methods that work and why they work.

Treating Conduct Disorders

Along with anxiety, conduct disorders have been found to be the most common problem among adolescents. Ironically, they're also the hardest to treat. How do you reach a teen who has lived his life with the deleterious effects of learning disorders or ADHD? An angry teen with no conscience? A teen who denies the fact that he has a problem?

Not with programs like Scared Straight. These have generated a lot of publicity, but follow-up studies have found that their results are only temporary, a superficial Band-Aid on problems that are deeply imbedded in the psyche of a delinquent teen. Scare tactics ultimately can't work on teenagers who feel omnipotent. "Yeah, well, I won't end up in jail," a delinquent will say defensively. Like cigarette smokers who deny their habit's hazards, these teens simply won't believe they'll wind up in prison—or worse.

Conduct-disordered teens need more than merely hearing about the dangers of their self-destructive paths. Like traveling down a deserted highway with a terrified driver, the treatment process delicately maneuvers between support and understanding, forcefulness and control. As outlined in *High Times/Low Times* by Dr. John E. Meeks, a good treatment program will:

- *Recognize the areas in which a CD teen excels and make sure he performs in those areas.* A boy who shows an interest in electronics should be encouraged to enroll in electronics courses at a trade school. Someone who seems mechanically inclined should be urged to pursue a career as a mechanic.
- *Try to build on weaknesses.* Whether it's improper social conduct

or a learning disability, a CD teen can be educated to better handle the stresses of everyday life.

- *Curb aggressive behavior with strict rules and restraints.* No matter what type of treatment program is employed, a positive set of stringent controls and guidelines will bring about a sense of self-worth and security in a CD patient.
- *Create a strong bond between therapist and patient.* A therapist can play a vital part in supplying the CD patient with a much-needed role model—someone the patient can have faith in—opening the door to recovery. But this trust does not come easily. The patient will test this relationship time and again through acting out, verbal abuse, and crime. It is the therapist's job to let the patient know that he does care for the patient, but that this type of behavior will not be tolerated.

This successful treatment process is achieved through a combination of six methods:

Individual therapy—which opens the lines of communication and trust between adolescent patient and adult therapist.

Cognitive/behavioral therapy—which concentrates on better ways to solve problems through step-by-step cognitive skill training.

Urge control—which develops through the strict enforcement of the rules within a hospital setting.

Moral development—which is fostered through insight therapy and skill-training workshops.

Medication—which is used to treat underlying depression, anxiety, and possible hyperactivity.

Family therapy—which recognizes conduct disorders as a family problem where no one is immune. Parents are taught new methods of management and discipline. They learn consistency and understanding. One method that has been proven to work are Parent Management Programs that use videotapes to instruct, train, and reinforce. Family therapy is crucial. Without cooperation and understanding within the entire family circle, the CD teen can fall back on his old ways when he leaves the hospital.

Later, I will be going over these and other treatment strategies in depth.

Conduct disorders are treatable. But it requires patience, understanding, and time. As one of our patients said, "When a lot of people first come here, to [Fair Oaks] and everything, they think that they don't have problems. I think that's one of the reasons why some people take longer at the hospital and have to have that more therapeutic environment. But I also think once you start working in the program, it's like you realize that you do have problems. And it's like all these things just start coming out—and you see that you really do have problems to work out, and that you're like glad you made the effort this time. You feel better about yourself."

There is hope for these troubled teens. And, better yet, there is real help.

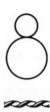

EATING DISORDERS

Roberta ate three apples, one bag of celery, several carrots, two pieces of bread spread with peanut butter, and half a container of yogurt every day.

She thought she was eating too much, so she increased her daily exercise from five miles of jogging to seven. She added two hours of calisthenics and three hundred laps a day in her family's swimming pool.

Roberta was always active. She was slightly overweight for her 5'5" height, but her mother always told her it was only "baby fat" and that she'd lose it when she grew up. Roberta began her period two years ago. At that time, she tried out for the girl's varsity basketball team at her private school. She didn't make it; her coach told her "to get into better shape and we'll see." That was all Roberta needed to hear. She started the excessive diet and exercise regime that would ultimately bring her to Fair Oaks Hospital.

But Roberta's story wasn't simply one of immediate cause and effect. Her transformation from a bright, normal girl into an anorexic was gradual and underneath her desire to be thin there were complicated family issues at work.

When Roberta was six, her family moved from Chicago to Atlanta. When she was ten, they left Atlanta and came to New Jersey. Roberta never fully adjusted to the moves. She had difficulty making new friends and, as she told me in our first interview, she never really felt that she "fit in." To make matters worse, her father, an executive in a prominent corporation, was never home. Over the years, he went from a middle-management position to a vice-presidency. Roberta claimed that her younger sister "reaped all the benefits." She said her parents treated her differently; they seemed to expect more from her because she was the oldest.

When Roberta stopped eating, the family problems exacerbated. She got into "raging battles" with her mother. "I lost seven pounds in one week once, and my mother was so angry." Roberta told me that her behavior gave her some control over her mother—who was always telling her what to wear, what to say, and how to act.

Things came to a head when Roberta injured her knee during one of her runs. The family doctor gave her strict instructions not to exercise for several weeks. Terrified that she'd gain back the pounds she'd lost, Roberta cut her caloric intake even further. Every day, she would eat only one bowl of farina, one carrot, two cans of diet soda, and eight bites of cold chicken. This led to severe carbohydrate cravings. On Saturday nights, when her parents were out, Roberta would binge on cookies, ice cream, and bowls of cold cereal. She would then make herself throw up. It was around this time that Roberta stopped menstruating.

The day after her parents discovered a stash of over-the-counter diet pills, laxatives, and diuretics, they brought her to Fair Oaks.

Roberta was suffering from an eating disorder. Her extreme diet and exercise program gave her one area to control in a life that felt overwhelming and powerless. The deprivation she experienced reinforced her feelings of worthlessness; she didn't deserve the gratification she derived from food. And the weight loss itself proved to be a vehicle of attention, of getting the nurturing she so sorely needed.

Before we could help Roberta with her depression and conflict, we had to build up her body. Before she entered the Adolescent Unit, she underwent a battery of tests. Her potassium was low; her heartbeat was barely audible. She showed all the symptoms of starvation. Roberta was fed intravenously at first; she slowly built up to solid foods that we coaxed her to eat. When the malnutrition disappeared, we began a treatment program consisting of family, group, and individual therapy—as well as medication to help her with her depressive symptoms.

She participated in the Performance Group and began to learn important social skills.

After ten months, Roberta was ready to go home. Her weight was once again within normal range. Her eyes were bright; she was energetic and hopeful. The relationship with her family improved and she was actually eager to go back to school. The last I heard, she had not only made the varsity basketball team—but she was also one of its stars.

GENERAL SYMPTOMS OF AN EATING DISORDER

- Intense fear of getting fat—which does not diminish with weight loss
- Emaciation
- Obsession with food and weight loss
- Stopped menstruation
- No known physical illness to account for weight loss
- Recurrent episodes of binge eating—consisting of large quantities of food consumed within two hours at least once a week for four weeks
- Awareness of abnormal eating patterns
- Fear of inability to stop eating during binge stage
- Depressed mood
- Self-deprecatory thoughts after binges
- Disturbed body image
- Self-induced vomiting
- Repeated bouts of losing weight through highly restrictive diets, vomiting, diuretics, or cathartics
- Willful starvation
- Excessive exercise

THE UNIQUE CHARACTERISTICS OF EATING DISORDERS

Dieting has become a national obsession—especially among women. In the 1920s, not one single article about dieting appeared in *Ladies' Home Journal, Good Housekeeping,* or *Harper's.* By 1980 there were 1.25 diet articles *per issue.* Other studies bear this out:

- In a *Glamour* magazine survey of 33,000 women, asking how they felt about their bodies and food, 41 percent said they were unhappy with their bodies—and 30 percent of them already weighed below established norms.

- Over the past twenty years, the weight of *Playboy* centerfolds has decreased significantly.
- Since 1970, the winners of Miss America pageants have weighed much less than the average contestant.
- Research from Melpomene, an institute on sports medicine for women, found that women consistently choose an ideal body shape that's 20 percent *under* the average weight.

This trend toward slimness exerts a powerful social pressure on women—but it's only half the story. "Thin is in" also reflects an underlying cultural factor that puts women at greater risk of developing an eating disorder. Even in today's world of sexual equality, boys and girls are still raised differently. Boys are pressured to achieve, to handle things for themselves. Girls, on the other hand, are encouraged more to ask for help—which translates into passivity and dependency. But, as they grow up and start school, girls are also encouraged to be autonomous and successful. They are expected to complete their education, to compete in the workplace—*and* to be a successful wife and mother. The delusion of "having it all" becomes a proliferation of "shoulds" and a pursuit of an elusive perfection—which adds further confusion to the "feminine," helpless role many women learn as children. The result is a fear of success and rejection—compounded by guilt for not being as "perfect" as a woman "should" be. In 1964 a study by Matina Horner found that 65 percent of college women both feared and avoided success. Ten years later that number rose to 88.2 percent. Today, many women are still faced with the conflicting drives between passivity, perfection, and independence. This ambiguity and confusion leaves many contemporary women vulnerable and insecure. In their quest for self-esteem and confidence, many of them turn to a more clear-cut area to control: their bodies.

For a girl approaching adolescence, these social and cultural conditions have even more implications. A young girl's body changes in puberty. She accumulates more body fat; she begins to sexually mature. Along with these hormonal and body-shape changes come new perceptions and new emotions—all of which focus on her body. It's easy for a young girl to react to this "brave new body" with exaggeration, exasperation, and even fear—especially because self-esteem, stability, and confidence are being redefined, tested, and developed during these adolescent years. Combined with the external pressures brought to bear from her school, her family, her friends, and from society at large, this exaggerated reaction can become a powder keg of emotion that explodes into an eating disorder.

The risk is even more insidious if this adolescent girl is white and from a high-income family. The Ten State Nutrition Survey, which studied over forty thousand people of all ages, proved that eating disorders are ten times more common in girls than boys—and that they hit this particular group the hardest. Here are their results:

- Girls tend to have more body fat than boys—at every age.
- As puberty approaches, both boys and girls gain weight. But during adolescence, boys lose weight, while girls accumulate more fat.
- "You can't be too rich or too thin" is a reality that begins early for many girls. During adolescence, girls in low-income families start out leaner, but end up fatter than girls in high-income homes—who make conscious efforts to lose weight.
- This same trend was seen among white and black girls, regardless of income. Black girls start their adolescence leaner than white girls, but end up with more body fat.

It's easy to see why models, athletes, and dancers are even more focused on their body shape—and why many of them develop eating disorders. To be lean means an athlete can run that extra mile. To be slender means a dancer can pirouette with grace. To be thin means a model can appear in the glossy pages of a fashion magazine. For these young adults, work and passion are tied up in their weight.

But what about the average girl? Not every Caucasian teenaged girl succumbs to an eating disorder—despite the pressures of adolescence. The reason some girls develop problems and others don't is more than a matter of society's social and cultural dictates. It is a complex combination of biology, psychology, and familial factors. Let's go over them now.

FAMILY TIES. On the surface, the parents of teens with eating disorders seem to be happy, stable, and well-adjusted. But, as studies show, this "Norman Rockwell" façade hides secret disillusionment and competition. Their parents can be overprotective—and preoccupied with appearances and success. They use their teen to "make up for" their own unfulfilled aspirations and dreams. In fact, an *over*involved mother and an *under*involved father with rigid expectations has been seen in 30 to 40 percent of the cases studied. My own experience bears these factors out: One of my patients at Fair Oaks, a girl from a well-to-do home, complained that her father was never home—but he was still the "boss." He set down strict rules that she and her brothers had to obey, including the time they woke up every morning, the grades they must achieve in school, and the manners they showed other people. Her father was always punishing her because, in her words, "I never measured up." Her mother, on the other hand, was overly solicitous. A woman who had given up her marketing career for her family, she had involved herself in every aspect of her children's lives. She continually interrupted her daughter during the first Fair Oaks interview to remind her of something she hadn't yet said. She raised her daughter's sleeve to show me a rash on her arm.

Eating disorders plug into the "open system" that was formulated by Dr. Salvador Minuchin. They discovered that in families that exhibited entanglement in each others' lives, overprotectiveness, rigidity, and lack of conflict resolution through such behavior as poor communication, these characteristics helped create and maintain a child's psychosomatic symptoms. These symptoms, in turn, maintained the family balance. By focusing, for example, on their teen's eating disorder, they could avoid open conflict. The family could submerge their hostilities and problems in their teenager—through overprotectiveness or blame. The teen and her eating disorder become the problem—and the family or marital conflicts that started it all are swept under the rug. Unfortunately, this not only perpetuates the eating disorder, but it makes the teen an active player in her parents' game of covert conflict and hostility. A study of anorexic teens found that as teenagers regained their normal weight through treatment, their parents' neuroses and problems worsened—especially if there were marital conflicts. Another study discovered that an anorexic patient slept poorly, agitated and aroused, whenever she was visited by her twin sister or mother.

Family history also plays a role. Studies have found that teens who develop eating disorders have alcoholism, drug abuse, or other poor impulse control disorders within the family sphere. In one particular study of 420 close relatives of 89 patients with eating disorders, Dr. James I. Hudson et al. discovered an increased risk of depression among all the family members. Whether this finding is a result of inherited genes or of inherited psychodynamic behavior, the fact is that disorders can be traced through the generations. Another one of my patients at Fair Oaks had a great-grandmother who had committed suicide and a grandmother who had an eating disorder and a major depression.

Given this backdrop, all that's needed to set the eating disorder "play" in motion is stress. As with the other disorders I've already discussed, the inability to cope with stress can result in an eating disorder. In fact, Drs. H.G. Morgan and G.F.M. Russell found that family stress preceded the disorder in 50 percent of the cases they studied. On the other hand, the stress of the eating disorder itself can cause family dysfunctioning.

In short, family ties can bind. But there are still two other arenas where eating disorders are staged, two settings that are intricately related.

THE PSYCHOLOGICAL FACTOR. Imagine this scenario: You are a young girl approaching adolescence. Perhaps your family never quite encouraged your expressions of individuality. Perhaps you've never developed your own sense of identity. Perhaps you've always wanted to please your parents, but you've never been sure what it is they really want. Instead, you've found yourself completely dependent on others for feelings of self-worth and confidence.

You're starting to feel frustrated, scared, and out of control. After all, you're fairly intelligent; you want to do well in school and please your parents. But as you get closer and closer to puberty, your body starts to change. People seem to expect more from you. Not just your parents, but your teachers in school, your friends—everybody seems to be burdening you with responsibility and rushing you into situations that make you feel uncomfortable. The demands and stresses of adolescence are becoming intolerable. As a child, you never quite separated from your parents, and, now, as adolescence repeats the "separation/individuation process" discussed in chapter one, it's almost too much to take. Here you are, experiencing this push of independence versus its concurrent and resentful pull of dependence on your parents, the strange ambiguity of surging sexual feelings—even your body is becoming unfamiliar and out of your control. It's no wonder you feel depressed. You simply don't want to grow up.

Maybe if you focused on your body, you'd feel better. Maybe the world would be a better place if you were thin. Maybe if your body stopped growing, you could stop these terrifying feelings and events.

You stop eating. Your body reacts, and this influences the way you think. Psychologically and physiologically, an eating disorder sets in—as does the third factor:

THE MIND/BODY CONNECTION. In many ways, teenagers are what they eat. Their growing bodies are regulated by processes at work in their brains—which are activated by the nutrients in the food they eat.

In medical terms, puberty involves the hypothalamic-anterior pituitary-gonadal axis. In real terms, the process goes something like this: Genetic transmissions, family cues, and other psychological messages are sent to the hypothalamus—an area of the brain that regulates appetite and weight gain. The hypothalamus is sensitive to these messages—especially when they are stressful, conflicted, and weighed down with the malnutrition that comes when a teen stops eating. The hypothalamus reacts by sending out a command to the anterior pituitary-gonadal areas of the body—which secrete growth hormones and influence sexual development. The order these glands receive from the hypothalamus is "imbalance your hormonal secretions." The result? Growth, especially sexual growth, is halted.

By not eating, a teen actually "switches off" the growth and sexual maturation that had so terrified her. At last, she can be in control of herself. And, as an added plus, she can remain the "perfect little girl" she assumes her parents want her to be. The longer a teenager stops eating, the greater the cognitive, emotional, and physical changes that occur and the more they react with one another:

- *Physically,* as we have seen, her entire growth process is thrown off-kilter. Her metabolism alters and slows, which helps her continue to refrain from eating. In fact, an anorexic girl displays the same symptoms victims of starvation show.
- *Cognitively,* her abstinence is reinforced by the "relief" she learned to feel when she "switched off" her growth.
- *Emotionally,* she shows symptoms of depression, including irritability, withdrawal, and feelings of self-loathing, which are only kept at bay with continued dieting. It makes sense that teenagers with eating disorders show the same endocrine dysfunction as those who are suffering from depression.

The eating disorder becomes her life. This girl has now created her own world—with no one in charge except herself.

As you can see, an eating disorder goes deeper than poor body image and constant dieting. As Drs. Paul L. Adams and Ivan Fras write in their book, *Beginning Child Psychiatry,* an eating disorder is "based on a disturbance of body image so severe that a morbid fear of gaining weight and becoming obese develops and, in turn, the normal function of eating becomes steeped in pathological signs and symptoms." There are two distinct types of disturbance, two dramas where an eating disorder can materialize: anorexia nervosa and bulimia nervosa. Let's go over them now.

Anorexia Nervosa

The key word here is emaciation. An anorexic teenager is painfully thin. She is probably in early adolescence, about to or just starting puberty. Her menstruation will have stopped. Like Roberta in our case study she will be compulsive and excessive about exercise. She will skip meals and, more often than not, be a high achiever at school. In fact, one out of every one hundred girls in English private schools are anorexics. These young girls are completely sold on their starvation and will not eat unless they are assured they will not gain weight. All their behavior and all their thoughts are directed toward losing weight. For example, when I asked Roberta what three wishes she would like to come true, she told me: "To never be fat, to be tall and beautiful," and, almost as an afterthought, "that there should never be a nuclear war."

ANOREXIA AND BULIMIA: HOW THEY ARE DIFFERENT— AND HOW THEY ARE THE SAME

	Anorexia	Bulimia
Emaciation	always present	absent
Drive for thinness	always present	variable
Behavior directed to weight loss	always present	variable
Bingeing	usually absent	always present
Vomiting	usually absent	always present
Laxative abuse	usually absent	usually present
Fear of fatness	present	always present
Normal weight or slight obesity	absent	always present
Periods	usually absent	present

Adapted from "An Overview of Eating Disorders" by L. K. George Hsu in *Basic Handbook of Child Psychiatry,* vol. 5, Joseph D. Noshpitz, editor-in-chief, et al. New York: Basic Books, Inc., 1987.

Though anorexia can include bingeing and purging episodes, they are much more prevalent in the second type of eating disorder, bulimia nervosa.

Bulimia Nervosa

Bulimia is five times more common than anorexia—and it can affect young women throughout their adolescence and beyond.

- 2.2 million women binge and purge on a weekly basis.
- Between 4.5 percent and 19 percent of U.S. college girls admit to being bulimic.
- A survey of three hundred women in an American shopping mall found that 10.3 percent had suffered from bulimia when they were teenagers—and half of them were still suffering.

Although bulimia literally means "ox appetite" in Greek, bulimic teens are usually at normal weight or slightly overweight. They desperately fear becoming fat; they don't want to be all skin and bones, but they are terrified of obesity. Usually suffering from an underlying dysthymic depression or anxiety, their self-image is nil—and completely tied up with their body image. Thus, they begin to diet. In fact, they will usually begin their bulimic cycle with an anorexic drive to lose weight. But this prolonged, severe dieting regime causes extreme cravings for carbohydrates—from junk food to pasta. The temptation soon proves overwhelming, and they are compelled to eat. The cycle begins:

1. Breaking their rigid "food rules," they take that first bite.
2. They immediately feel a sense of overwhelming release, pleasure, and abandon.
3. They give themselves up to this liberating force, literally eating as if there was no tomorrow, consuming up to several thousand calories within one binge. It can last for minutes or hours—and occur up to ten times a day.
4. But, sooner or later, the pleasure is stopped by a sense of intolerable guilt over losing control. The overwhelming fear of fatness takes hold. There is only one thing to do: purge through laxatives, diuretics, or vomiting—or by a combination of the three.
5. The purging over, these bulimic teens feel better. They make a new resolve to "start fresh." They begin their rigid dieting all over again—until the next craving to binge.

This binge/purge cycle is a coping mechanism for these teenaged girls. It relieves their tension and balances their two conflicting emotions: to be slim and in control versus the freedom to eat as many forbidden foods as they want. They don't want to vomit, but they see no other way to stop weight gain.

Bulimics function well at school and at work, but they are more intolerant of stress. They suffer from mood swings. When they feel in control of their weight and are in the process of dieting, they feel good. When they feel the desire to binge, they become irritable and depressed. In short, they become prisoners of their binge/purge cycle. When it is firmly entrenched, their life *is* the cycle—and they see no way out.

Anorexia nervosa might be getting more press these days, but its roots go back to the Middle Ages. In 1225 the Bishop of Lincoln sent fifteen clerics to observe firsthand a Leicester nun who supposedly ate nothing but the eucharist for seven years. They stayed by her bedside for fifteen days—and confirmed the rumors. In the fourteenth century, a saint named Liduine of Schiedam supposedly dined on "a little piece of apple the size of a holy wafer."

Religious figures were not the only ones. In 1542 a physician wrote of a ten-year-old girl named Margaret Weiss who didn't eat for three years, but she still was "walking about, laughing, and talking like other children."

From "Anorexia Nervosa: History and Psychological Concepts" by Michael Strober, *Handbook of Eating Disorders,* ed. Kelly D. Brownell and John P. Foreyt. New York: Basic Books, I.

Treating Eating Disorders

An eating disorder is very much a physiological illness—and both its psychological and physical symptoms must be treated. Malnutrition is a real problem. As we have seen, its physical effects reinforce the psychological problems. If a teenager is severely anorexic, she must be hospitalized and, if necessary, fed intravenously. Once her body is stronger, the eating disorder and its underlying depression or anxiety can be treated—through medication and individual, family, and cognitive skill training therapy.

Unfortunately, therapy is easier said than done. Teens suffering from anorexia or bulimia are usually very resistant. They don't want to be helped. They have created a world they can control, and they don't want to give that up. Their fear of fatness, their poor body image, and their self-loathing are so ingrained and tied together that a therapist must use a great deal of patience and understanding to reach them. Because family dysfunction is such a strong factor in the development of an eating disorder, hospitalization is usually recommended. Within the security and boundaries of the hospital's walls, a teenager can learn to cope better with stress before returning home. She can build up her confidence and her self-image and separate her sense of worth from her body.

A teenager in a Performance Group audience once wrote: "Eating disorders: Not liking yourself and then not eating, and eventually eating, then feeling worse about yourself. A never-ending cycle." It doesn't have to be this way. An eating disorder can be cured. The cycle can be stopped. I know. I have seen hundreds of adolescents with eating disorders who have been helped at Fair Oaks Hospital—and who have gone on to full, productive lives.

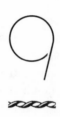

ANXIETY DISORDERS

Casey's mother told me her daughter was always worried about something. In school it was her grades. At home it was her friends and a phone that never rang for her. Casey was only comfortable hanging out with her parents—and she was sure no one else liked her.

When Casey was admitted to Fair Oaks Hospital she suffered from seizures for no apparent neurological or physiological reason. As a child she had had fierce temper tantrums, knocking her head against a wall and crying. Now, she would roll over on the floor, biting her fingers and moaning, exhibiting a "pseudoseizure" behavior.

"I don't want to be this way, please help me," Casey said during her admissions interview. Tall and slender, she was an extremely bright fourteen-year-old girl with a high I.Q. She did well in school and had several close friends. Her childhood development was normal; she was equally adept at piano playing, English, and math. The problems began one afternoon at school; she had had a fight with a girlfriend. Casey was upset because she hadn't been invited to her house "like everyone else." Her girlfriend told her that she was going to invite her, but she hadn't yet seen Casey that day. Casey didn't believe her. They began to argue. Casey came home in tears.

Her mother was equally upset. She listened to Casey and tried to comfort her. But the next day, Casey didn't want to go to school. Her mother let her stay home. The next day, it happened again. This time, Casey's mother insisted she go. Casey agreed—if she didn't have to take the school bus. She didn't want to see her girlfriend. Her mother once again agreed; she drove Casey to school. On the way, Casey had her first pseudoseizure. Frightened, her mother took her to the family doctor—who could find nothing wrong.

The next day, Casey waited until the other kids went inside; only then would she get out of the car. This went on for a week. The following Monday, Casey put her foot on the car's accelerator as her mother approached the school. Her mother began screaming. Casey had her second pseudoseizure. For the next several months, Casey was shunted back and forth from specialist to specialist until, finally, she came to Fair Oaks.

When I interviewed her, I discussed her childhood; I did a lifeline profile to determine where her stress—and her inability to cope—began. Casey had suffered from asthma ever since she was four years old. She also had a great many allergies when she was young. When she was growing up, she couldn't eat the ice cream and cake the other children could at various birthday parties. She felt like an "outsider"—which was reinforced when her parents sent her to sleepaway camp one summer. Casey was miserable; she cried almost nonstop and her parents were forced to bring her home within two weeks.

This pervasive feeling of abandonment and rejection continued during the school year. Though she had friends, Casey never felt comfortable with them. She was sure they were talking about her; she was sure they didn't really like her.

Her problems were compounded by family difficulties. Casey's brother suffered from congenital heart problems; he was in and out of hospitals. "He always gets more attention than me," Casey said. Further, as a salesman for a manufacturing firm, Casey's father had to relocate three times in six years. He was rarely home, but Casey said she would "die if anything happened to him." She spent much time with her mother, who had become depressed. The moves, the problems with her son, her anxiety over Casey—all had taken their toll. "We always gave in to Casey's tantrums. It seemed easier," Casey's mother told me. But now she treated her daughter with trepidation. "I never know when she's going to explode and have another seizure." Consequently, the atmosphere in Casey's home was tense. This family dysfunction, combined with Casey's childhood illnesses, her inability to separate from her parents, and her inability to cope with the stresses involved in adolescence, proved much too much. All Casey needed was one more incident to put her "over the edge." The fight with her girlfriend provided the catalyst for the pseudoseizures to begin—a manipulative defense against an anxiety that had become too much to bear.

Casey suffered from a severe anxiety disorder. She was terrified of not being liked or accepted. She was terrified that her parents might leave her—even as she wished for independence. In short, she was afraid of growing up.

At Fair Oaks, Casey was put on medication to treat her anxiety and her underlying depression. We showed her relaxation techniques to help her cope whenever she felt a seizure coming on. Cognitive therapy helped her see her fears and insecurities in a more rational manner. Individual, group, and family therapies encouraged Casey to gain insight into her problems; they helped promote better communications within her family circle. Finally, social skills training, including participation in the Performance Group, helped Casey find confidence in herself. Today, Casey is learning to accept who she is. She has not had a pseudoseizure in five months. She has gone back to school—and she takes the bus every day.

The Symptoms of Anxiety Disorders

The following symptoms are general signs of anxiety only. If your teen exhibits two or more of them for a period longer than two weeks, it can mean that he or she is suffering from one of several different types of anxiety disorder. Consult your family physician for an accurate diagnosis.

- Complaints of chest pains or aches
- Diarrhea and frequent upset stomachs
- Difficulty concentrating
- Dizziness
- Eyelid or facial twitches
- Little energy
- Headache complaints
- Fearful behavior
- Impatience
- Sleep problems
- Crankiness and irritability

- Shortness of breath
- Trembling or shaking
- Overanxiety in leaving parents
- Overanxiety in leaving the house
- Rituallike behavior, including too many showers or too much focus on neatness
- A general nervousness that has lasted for over six months

THE UNIQUE CHARACTERISTICS OF ANXIETY DISORDERS

On the television show "The Wonder Years," actor Fred Savage's eleven-year-old character, Kevin, often finds himself embroiled in anxiety-producing situations. From avoiding the strangleholds of the school bully and trying to win the heart of his girl, Winnie, to coping with his family's eccentricities, Kevin has his hands full. He gets worried and he gets confused. But, by the end of the show's half-hour format, he has always learned a valuable lesson on life.

Although Kevin is make-believe, his situations are not. We can all remember the pain when a friend rejected us, the worry we experienced before a test, and the fear we felt when the principal confronted us. In adolescence, bouts of anxiety are as normal as feeling depressed occasionally. But, as with depression, if a teen's anxiety lasts longer than a few weeks, it can signal a problem—with a life of its own.

Contrary to the jargon of the day, anxiety is not simply "free-floating." Anxiety in adolescence falls into four distinct categories, each with its own theme, its own motivation, and its own characteristics.

Separation-Anxiety Disorder

"People who need people" includes us all. To be human means to form attachments. We are a social species, interrelating with others and developing interdependency from the moment we are born. And, because the very first person who nurtures us is usually our mother, the way that relationship develops becomes crucial to the way we later relate to others in the world at large.

Separation and individuation is an important process in the development of self. As we saw in chapter one, this process begins in what Margaret Mahler called the "rapprochement stage." Here, a toddler begins to recognize his own separateness from his mother—but he is still not ready to stand alone. He will be motivated to explore his new world, but he will also want to make sure mom is standing by.

This can be a difficult time for children. The more aware a child becomes of his individuality, the more anxiety he will feel. To lose that omnipotent bond, that feeling of "oneness" between himself and her mother, is necessary—but it is also scary.

Alone, this anxiety would be enough to complicate a child's universe, but aggression, which is the fuel that energizes the motivation to separate in the first place, makes matters worse. Together, this anxiety and aggression combination can promote the development of a healthy and separate individual. Or it can or create the feeding ground for problems that crop up when adolescence begins, and the "separation and individuation" process is repeated in the context of the outside world.

Love always involves risk. Because attachments are so vital to us we inevitably fear losing them. But healthy development keeps those fears within limits. When a mother is sensitive to her child's needs, balancing encouragement with security, her child can cope with his complex feelings. His aggression becomes internalized, strengthening his new, burgeoning self; his anxiety subsides as he continues to grow. But, when a mother is not available, his aggressive impulses are fraught with anxiety that won't go away. The fear of loss becomes overwhelming. He simply cannot leave his mother, because he fears he will lose her love.

This situation is more common than you might think. A lot of kids get stuck trying to get something from their parents that they are never going to get. They keep looking for approval, for security, for a guarantee that love will last forever. A case in point is the thirty-year-old woman who still calls her mother to ask her which dress she should buy—or the thirty-two-year-old man who can't leave home.

When the fear of losing a parent's love becomes excessive, a separation-anxiety disorder can emerge, usually in combination with depression. A 1985 study of fifty-nine five- to sixteen-year-olds with major depression found that 86 percent of the prepuberty group and 47 percent of the postpuberty group also met the criteria for separation-anxiety disorder. Its specific symptoms, as listed in the DSM-III-R, include a child's:

- *Unrealistic worry* that his parents will eave or be harmed.
- *Fear of being lost,* hurt, killed, or kidr.apped.
- *Reluctance to go to school* in order to stay home with his parents. Unfortunately, many parents think their child's problems are solved when he or she returns to the school environment. But this isn't necessarily true. Joanie, an eleven-year-old girl suffering from separation-anxiety disorder, did indeed go back to school—as long as she could sleep in her parents' bedroom every night.
- *Unwillingness to sleep away from his parents.*
- Avoidance of solitary pursuits.
- Anxiety dreams about separation.
- *Physical symptoms,* including dizziness, stomachaches, headaches, and chills. A child will usually display physical symptoms rather than verbalizing his fears—especially in adolescence—where admitting he wants to be with his parents is embarrassing and he must save face.
- *Emotional distress* when a separation draws near.
- *Inability to work or play* unless his parents are around.

But there is more to separation anxiety than these symptoms show. Separation anxiety disorder is a two-way street involving parent and child. A study of eleven emotionally disturbed nursery school children found that as the children began moving away from their mothers to the play area, the mothers would move closer—intruding on their play to wipe noses or fix pant cuffs.

As this study proves, separation can be as difficult for the mother as for the child. A mother who doesn't trust babysitters outside the family circle, who constantly warns her child of the hazards and dangers outside the home, who "smothers" her child with overprotectiveness, is as bad as the mother who ignores her child during the "separation and individuation" process.

Overprotectiveness can spring from a mother who:

- *Has her child late in life, especially after years of infertility.* The mother of one of my patients had tried for so long to have a child that she couldn't let go. She had been so focused on getting pregnant that her baby literally was her life.
- *Wants to protect her child from the unhappy childhood experiences that she herself had.* Another mother had been the victim of abuse. She had been the pawn in a violent custody battle, and she had

vowed that her own children would never feel the fear, the shame, and the pain that she had experienced—or *any* negative emotions at all.

- *Experienced the problems of separation and individuation when she was growing up.* I remember one woman who would not move out of her parents' neighborhood. Her son was always at his grandparents' house. When the woman's father died, she felt the same fears of abandonment she'd felt when she was young—and she communicated those fears to her child.

- *Turns to her child for the only secure relationship in a bad marriage.* One particular woman was contemplating divorce when her husband died in an accident. She became guilt-ridden, anxious, and depressed, irrationally believing that if she did not constantly watch out for her daughter, she too would come to harm just as her husband did. The child soon picked up on her mother's fears. She became terrified of the outside world, especially when her mother wasn't around. Neither of them could let go of the other.

In addition to overprotectiveness, another factor in separation-anxiety disorders is hostile dependency. When a mother is in a bad marriage, she might displace her anger from her husband onto her child—or she might feel tied down by her child and resent her. Angry thoughts, no matter how normal at times, can make many a mother feel guilty—which will make her cling even more to her child. The child, in turn, becomes hostile, because she senses this anger, and she cannot totally trust her parents. She then might cry or throw temper tantrums or, like Casey, act out with pseudoseizures in an effort to control her parents. In fact, when children bargain and threaten a great deal to get what they want, they can actually begin to display the characteristics of conduct disorders.

Unfortunately, a child's temper tantrums make parents even more resentful. They feel even more guilt, which, in turn, will make them act more overprotectively—and the cycle of hostile dependency continues, tightening this unhealthy symbiotic bond.

Overanxious Disorder of Adolescence

Fear. That rush of adrenaline that flows through our system. Faster heartbeat, muscular contractions, rapid breathing. The activated nervous, cardiovascular, and glandular "all systems go" designed to make us ready for "fight or flight."

In prehistoric times, this adrenaline rush was a welcome weapon, a biological way to prepare to meet an angry animal or an aggressive neighboring tribe. By the time the emergency was over, the adrenaline, the faster heartbeat, and the rapid breathing would dissipate, and things would quiet down—until the next danger came along.

But today, that adrenaline rush often has nowhere to go. When confronted with a stressful situation, we experience that same fear our ancestors did—but we are not about to use the surge of power for "fight or flight." A boy is not going to knock down a teacher for making him take a surprise quiz. A girl is not going to hit her boyfriend because he didn't ask her out for Saturday night. Instead of concrete danger like wild animals and murderous enemies, today's dangers are more internal and more ambiguous. Instead of fear, we feel anxiety—an *anticipated* threat to our own individual security or safety, which can mean anything from an irrational boss to a phone call that never comes.

Learning to cope with anxiety is a lonely business. We must learn ways to cope with conflict and stress, ways that are unique to our own life experiences and history. Depending on the intensity of the feeling of anxiety itself, the extremity of the provoking situation, and the health of one's psychological development, a person can either be free from anxiety most of the time—or constantly living with it. Without good coping skills, this anxiety becomes chronic—regardless of what situations a person is forced to face. In teens, this chronic anxiety can result in an anxiety disorder. Teens who suffer from it are:

- *Anxious about every situation and every person they meet.* They are worrywarts, excessively preoccupied about possible accidents, school performance, athletic prowess, and popularity.
- *High-strung, nervous, and lacking in emotional security.* They are unhappy and need too much reassurance from their family, their teachers, and their peers.
- *Sickly and overly concerned about physical injury*—a stance often used to avoid participating in outside activities.
- *Prone to nightmares and irrational fears.* Their anxiety will interfere with their learning abilities; they simply cannot concentrate on the task at hand.
- *Restless*—constantly pulling at their hair, chewing on their nails, or exhibiting facial tics.
- *Usually found in more upper-class households* than teens with separation-anxiety disorders. Both boys and girls are equally susceptible.

- *Prone to phobias, panic attacks, and compulsive-obsessional behavior* (which I will discuss in detail later on in this chapter.)

Learning healthy ways to deal with conflict and stress begins at home. Parents who are inconsistent, neglectful, or overly critical can tax a child's coping abilities to the limit. Sometimes even one stressful life situation—the birth of another sibling, a move to another state, a family fight—can cause a child to develop an anxiety disorder.

It is true that in the same way parents communicate positive emotions to children, they also communicate uncertainty and worry. A girl I treated for an overanxious disorder came from a wealthy family that suddenly had to cut back when her father lost his job. Their economic problems were heightened by discord, conflicts, and worry over money. Her father began to drink, and this girl became extremely anxious. She counted the liquor bottles in the bar constantly; she was worried that her father's drinking would increase. She cut back on school lunches. When her parents started to argue, she would go in her room and close the door. She would sit on the edge of her bed, rocking back and forth, moaning. She became her parents' "fear barometer." The more worried and upset they became, the more her anxious symptoms would increase.

But anxious mothers do not automatically raise anxious children. Studies have found that children of anxious or insecure mothers will not become overly fearful themselves as long as their mother's insecurity is not coupled with hostility. Other studies have found, however, that children of mothers suffering from major depression are at greater risk for developing an overanxious disorder.

As with any illness, it's important to know that your teenager's overanxious disorder is not something else. A learning disorder, for instance, can make a child anxious about school. Family dysfunction can breed anxiety, as can anemia, malnutrition, and substance abuse. But if your teen has been consistently and generally anxious for over six months and there is no physical cause or any other underlying psychological disorder, she or he can be suffering from an overanxious disorder of adolescence.

Obsessive-Compulsive Disorder

Jaynie opens and closes each door six times before she can enter or leave a room

Bill has seven pairs of shoes, one of which he has assigned to each day of the week. He will only wear his sneakers on Monday, his loafers on Tuesday, his black shoes on Wednesday. . . .

Hamilton insists on being the first kid in class. If he somehow doesn't make it between bells, he refuses to go inside the classroom.

Rosemary follows George around school all day. She continues to call him every single night, even though he's told her he doesn't want to see her anymore. She knows he doesn't love her, but she can't help it.

These teenagers are suffering from obsessive-compulsive disorder, an illness that may strike up to 10 percent of all children. From being afraid to take a shower in gym class to finding a kiss repulsive, from excessive hand washing to repeating a silent prayer countless times a day, this disorder not only causes pain within its victims, it interferes with all areas of development and growth. Boys will show its symptoms around nine and a half years old; the onset for girls is usually eleven.

All young children use "magical thinking" to some extent to relieve anxiety. They will wish they can erase the ink they spilled on the carpet. They will hope their parents won't get sick. But, eventually, they realize this magic doesn't work and learn other ways to cope with their fears.

Some teens become compulsive in only one aspect of their lives. Whether they become computer wizards, astronomy or meteorology experts, or simply memorize every TV show from the 1950s, their compulsion with their special interest can create havoc with their friendships and in their families—but this doesn't necessarily mean that they are obsessive-compulsive. Compulsions or obsessions are often a normal, transitory part of a child's development Given time, children usually overcome them. The boy who memorizes every TV show soon forgets what he learned when he goes to college. The computer wizard gets a scholarship to a top-notch university and finds both personal and professional success.

A true obsession-compulsion starts with an intrusive idea (obsession) or impulse (compulsion) that fills a child with dread. He feels powerless to stop his thoughts or his urges; he becomes guilt-ridden, anxious, and scared. In his desire to stop his obsessions or compulsions, he will make up elaborate rules and rituals that temporarily keep his anxiety at bay. But, ultimately, he cannot ease his pain. Caught in an unending maze of desire and resistance, the compulsions and obsessions become his life. He becomes, literally, a slave. He doesn't want to step on the cracks in the sidewalk, but he has no choice. If he doesn't, his father might die.

She doesn't want to button and unbutton her shirt ten times, but it's the only way she can keep her sexual feelings from being exposed. Like the scientist in the science-fiction movie *Forbidden Planet,* these teens are terrified that their worst nightmares, their worst thoughts and desires, will come true.

It makes sense that obsessive-compulsives are profoundly unhappy. They are humorless and unenthusiastic and they believe they are always right. They are also verbose in a pedantic, "stuffed shirt" way. And they learn to act the way they do from their parents—their first role models. In fact, a study by the National Institute of Mental Health found that 20 percent of obsessive-compulsive teens had a family history of the disorder. These parents:

- *Are highly verbal.* They use talk as if it has some mythical power to erase dark thoughts. Consequently emotions are ignored or talked away.
- *Do not prize warm relationships.* They have few close friends and they don't encourage their children to seek out friends.
- *Usually hoard money.* They will spend a great deal of time on saving and accounting.
- *Have very rigid, set rules.* They don't abide unacceptable behavior in their children. Unfortunately, the message their children receive is this: Parental love is based on meeting strict, perfect standards and the slightest infringement means rejection—and a terrifying loss of love. Anger toward their parents builds—which leads to guilt. Combined with trying to live up to an impossible standard, these forces help create an obsessive-compulsive disorder.

Panic Attacks and Phobias

When anxiety builds up, it needs an outlet. When a teen is unable to cope with stress, he won't be open to deep breathing or a run around the block. Instead, the anxiety continues to build—until it finds a destructive outlet: a panic attack.

One stressful life situation can set off a panic attack, but so can a series of "trivial" events one right after the other—a bad mark on a test, a family argument, a parking ticket, a dateless Saturday night. Stress alone, however, does not a panic attack make. Recent research has found that people can be biologically predisposed to anxiety and panic. As Dr. Mark S. Gold explains in *The Good News About Panic, Anxiety, and Phobias,* chemical reactions in the brain can trigger anxiety.

POST-TRAUMATIC SHOCK DISORDER (PTSD)

Discovered during the Vietnam War, this condition causes much pain in its victims. From physical distress to depression, people suffering from PTSD are literally haunted by a trauma that never dies. For adolescents, that trauma could be the death of a parent, a divorce, or even a move to a new town. The result is pain, panic, and possible regression. Some children forget certain language skills. They can forget their socialization development, reverting back to the "safe" days of infancy—forgetting personal grooming habits and even their toilet training. PTSD might be more prevalent in adolescence than initially thought. A 1985 study of fifteen Vietnam vets suffering from PTSD versus eleven vets who showed no symptoms discovered that the ones who succumbed to PTSD had been teenagers in Vietnam, developing young adults who had formed an intense attachment to their buddies.

The nerve cell body in the brain called the locus coeruleus has one main function: to manufacture stimulating chemicals called catecholamines. Other nearby nerve endings balance the catecholamine activity by releasing self-tranquilizing chemicals. But sometimes there are too many catecholamines. Sometimes the ones that are there are extremely hyperactive. And sometimes the other nerve endings aren't working up to par—and the tranquilizing chemicals can't do their job. Consequently, the stimulating catecholamines move about unchecked—to trigger anxiety.

More proof: Thanks to a sophisticated technique called positron emission tomography (P.E.T.), scientists have been able to peer into the brain's inner workings. When they examined the brains of people who were having panic attacks, they found an abnormal flow of blood in the parahippocampalgyrus, a region of the brain associated with emotional expression and fear.

Like depression, panic attacks have a biological component. In fact, many teens who suffer from panic disorders also suffer from major depression. In a study of sixty-one adolescents, 24 percent were found to suffer from panic attacks and 24.5 percent from major depression. Another study found that seven out of ten cases of teens with panic disorders also have a higher rate of depression. They feel guilty. They lose interest in things. They are filled with anxiety. And they lose weight.

Panic attacks usually begin between the ages of fifteen and nineteen—and they can be the most debilitating effect of anxiety. A teen in the throes of a panic attack will feel dizzy and faint. She will have difficulty breathing; she will begin to sweat and her heart will pound. She will be terrified that she will die. Though panic attacks can be a symptom associated with separation anxiety, overanxious disorders, and obsessive-compulsive disorders, it can also trigger a different disorder: a phobia. When a teen has a panic attack in a certain situation, he may begin to associate the situation with panic. If he had an attack in the middle of the night, he can become afraid of the dark. If she had an attack in English class, she can become afraid to go to school.

Every child has fears. One study found that 90 percent of the children they sampled had at least seven fears. Another study, discussed in *Principles and Practice of Child Psychiatry* by Drs. Stella Chess and Mahin Hassibi, found that sex and socioeconomic factors influence the fears that children have:

- Lower-class boys fear violence with knives and guns
- Higher-class boys fear car accidents and disasters
- Lower-class girls fear strangers and animals
- Higher-class girls fear kidnapping and shipwrecks

These single-object phobias are called simple phobias and they range from fear of elevators to fear of bees.

But fear is not phobia. A child's fears are a reflection of his limited scope and understanding; they depend on a specific age or stage of development. As he grows up, the object of his fears become more abstract. Fear of the dark is replaced with fear of death or burglars. Eventually, the fears disappear or become a part of his memory. But when these fears take over a child's life, dominating his feelings, his thoughts, and his behavior, they become phobias. And if this youngster is forced to face the object of his fear, he will experience anxiety and terrifying panic.

Phobias don't go away with time. They have nothing to do with a child's age or development. As with panic attacks, a stressful life event can trigger them. In fact, in a study of thirty-five school-phobic children, a physical illness, a parental separation, or a parental depression occurred in the year before the phobia began.

Complex phobias are more abstract than simple phobias. They involve situations, people, and environments. School and social phobias are the two most common complex phobias among teens. Let's briefly go over them now.

SCHOOL. When a teen starts junior high, she can become overwhelmed with its more impersonal structure, its added responsibility, and its strange new faces. If she is not ready to become more independent, if she is struggling with her new feelings of aggression and sexuality, or if she simply needs more support, this new school environment can be terrifying. A case in point is John, the overindulged and spoiled baby of his family. Everyone thought John was cute—from his parents to his teachers. In school, he would "act out," but in adorable ways, and he was never reprimanded. Because he was so smart, he got good grades without a lot of studying. But when John started junior high, things changed. Three of his seventh-grade teachers insisted on hard work and nightly homework. They didn't appreciate his sense of humor, and they refused to indulge him. But John couldn't just stop his behavior; he simply didn't know how. He suddenly found school a place of embarrassment, a place where he was criticized and punished, where his very identity was under attack. He saw failure instead of his usual success and he refused to go. He believed that if he went to school he would die.

Teens with school phobias come from all different types of families—and there is no evidence to suggest that their parents are antisocial, abusive, or less involved in their child's activities than other parents. The children themselves are more emotionally dependent. They seek the security of home sweet home to cope with the stress of growing up. Some researchers actually consider school phobia the adolescent's agoraphobia, an adult fear of leaving the house. But adults know their phobias are not rational—even though they are powerless to stop them. Unfortunately, teens are not as developed. They truly believe that they will die or be injured if they face their phobic fear—which makes teenage phobics much more difficult to treat.

SOCIAL PHOBIAS. Being ridiculed or laughed at. Being robbed or bullied. Being called a "nerd." Being forced to stand up in front of a class and perform. Being seen naked in a gym class shower. All of these situations conjure up fear for many teens. The anticipation of shame, terror, or humiliation inhibits them from participating in any social activities. And, as in the case of "performance anxiety," if a teen is forced to recite something in an assembly, he will have a panic attack.

Why social phobia? A teen might not be able to cope with his sexual development. He might be uncomfortable with his new assertiveness and drive for independence. He might feel guilty about "leaving" his parents. He is terrified of losing the security he had at home. Everything inside him says, "I'm not ready for this!" If he has already been ridiculed in a social situation, his anxiety can become phobic. He associates a school dance or a club meeting with panic. He can't go through the pain again—or he will die.

As with the other adolescent disorders, many of these different anxiety disorders overlap. A separation anxiety can become an overanxious disorder. A school phobia can be a symptom of separation anxiety. The anxiety itself can be a symptom of an underlying major depression.

But whatever you call it, an anxiety disorder can debilitate—and harm a teenager's development. In fact, studies have found that teens who have overanxious disorders develop general anxiety as adults. Obsessive-compulsive teens become obsessive-compulsive adults. Unfortunately, teens suffering from anxiety are not always helped. As Dr. A. M. Graziano said, "Adults seem to minimize the importance of children's fears and to view such fears as a common, expected, transitory, and thus not particularly serious part of normal development."

Treating an anxiety disorder is almost an emergency situation. The longer a teenager feels fear and panic, the more fixed her defenses will be—and the harder the disorder will be to overcome. Anxiety must not be ignored or dismissed. To be forearmed is to be forewarned. Recognizing its symptoms is the first step; the second is getting proper help. If your teenager's anxiety is hurting him, there is treatment that can stop it in its tracks.

The Curtain Raiser: Treating Anxiety Disorders

Treating anxiety means teaching teenagers better ways to cope with stress. It means helping them develop confidence and a sense of security within themselves. It means understanding, patience, and support while using:

- *Cognitive therapy* to logically and systematically ease distorted, illogical thinking.
- *Psychotherapy* to help a teen gain insight into her mistrust, her fear of death and separation, and her anger.
- *Pharmaceuticals* to treat any underlying depression and any obsessive-compulsive behavior.
- *Behavior modification* to gradually expose a teen to his phobias—

and help him overcome them. If, for example, he is afraid to go to school, a therapist might have him go only to certain classes a few hours a week at a time.

- *Family therapy* to help everyone within the family circle understand the dynamics of the teen's anxiety—and to help parents resolve their own separation-anxiety or any other anxiety disorder.
- *Remedial schoolwork* to help a teen keep up with his grades if he is suffering from a school phobia.
- *Relaxation training* to teach a teen how to cope better with stress. Self-hypnosis, meditation, exercise, and deep breathing are all used to help calm anxiety.
- *Hospitalization,* if necessary, to provide a supportive atmosphere without any distractions.

We have now gone over the most common disorders found in adolescence. But there is one area we have yet to cover. It is the final cry for help, the result of a downward spiral that has been ignored or neglected. It is the ultimate culmination of a teenager's pain. It is suicide—and it too can be prevented.

SUICIDE

"I tried to kill myself." Five short words. One simple statement of fact. A universal plea that has brought more teenagers to Fair Oaks Hospital than any other disorder. Sixteen-year-old Ellen was no exception. She had tried to commit suicide four times in the past year. The first time she thought she was pregnant. She was so upset that she wrote a note: "I did not do my homework and I didn't wash my hair." She took twenty-two aspirins before she went to sleep, "fully expecting to die." The next morning, she woke up and discovered she had her period. She decided she loved life and she didn't want to kill herself anymore.

The second time, Ellen slit her wrists. "But it was superficial and I didn't tell anyone." It was the summer she began wearing braces on her teeth and special orthopedic shoes to correct a foot problem. "I felt so ugly. I felt so out of it."

Attempt number three involved eight sleeping pills, which Ellen stole from her mother. According to Ellen, she had gone to a party and came home drunk. "But I never drank a lot and it was the first time I ever did that." Her mother was furious and began screaming at her. After grabbing the pills, Ellen ran out of the house and went to a friend's home. She confided what she had done to her friend—who told her mother. Her friend's mother told Ellen's mother, who, in turn, insisted that Ellen see a therapist. Ellen agreed—as long as she could stay with her friend for a week.

The fourth suicide attempt was the result of an argument Ellen had with her mother. "My mother expects me to do everything and be an adult—but then she'll treat me like a child." It was snowing. Ellen walked out of the house with a knife. She slashed her wrists and watched her blood drip on the cold, white front stoop. "I realized I needed help. But I had to get out of my house."

She was brought to Fair Oaks Hospital that evening.

Ellen's story began when she was in eighth grade. It was then that her father lost his job. Severely depressed, he began sleeping twenty hours a day. He barely spoke to anyone and, when he did say anything, it was usually abusive. He began to drink. "It was like living with a dead person," Ellen told me in our first interview. She claimed that he would become furious if people were coming over. One time he ripped the phone out of the wall because he hated its ring. Ellen's mother was forced to go back to her nursing career. She began to work almost around the clock. When she wasn't working, she was crying. She relied more and more on Ellen to take care of her two younger brothers. Soon Ellen was cooking, cleaning, and managing the house.

But Ellen was still a child with much growing up to do. She learned to hate her father, a stranger who showed her no love or interest. She resented her mother for "putting up with him and not doing anything." She began to rely more and more on her friends—but she never really felt as if she belonged with them either. Ellen lived in a wealthy Connecticut suburb, but her family's bad financial straits made her uncomfortable. Her friends all had more money that she did; she couldn't participate in many of their activities. "I didn't fit in anymore."

The stress began to take its toll. Ellen's grades, which had always been excellent, began to slip. She began to overeat; she stopped caring about her appearance. She began dating a boy who took advantage of her. After he'd slept with her, he dropped her. When Ellen's period was late, thoughts of suicide consumed her days. She wanted help. She needed help. But she wasn't getting any. She took the twenty-two aspirins and the year of suicide attempts began.

Like half of all suicide victims, Ellen was suffering from a major depression—caused by the ongoing trauma of her family's dysfunction combined with the developmental stress arising from adolescence. Ellen really didn't want to kill herself; she just wanted to change things. It became her only way to cope with a world that held no hope.

At the Fair Oaks Adolescent Unit, Ellen was put on antidepressants. She participated in individual and group therapy; her family met twice weekly for family therapy. She became involved in the Performance Group; she participated in social skill training and, under the counseling of one of the hospital's registered dietitians began a weight-loss program.

Slowly, Ellen began to improve. She gained confidence and her self-esteem grew. She and her family learned to communicate in a more open manner. After eight months of hospitalization, Ellen was no longer depressed. She could go home. After all, she was young—and the world was full of promise.

Symptoms of Suicidal Thoughts or Actions

Unfortunately, there are no crystal balls, no magic oracles, and no one apt description that can accurately pinpoint a teen who might try to commit suicide. But there are specific warning signs that signal trouble, specific stress-filled situations that bring pain, confusion—and a possible suicide attempt. Because suicide is usually the harrowing result of a depression that has gone out of control, suicidal symptoms are very similar to those of depression disorders. Here are these "red flag" symptoms and situations. If your teen exhibits any of them, he might not attempt suicide—but he will need your help. The more warning signs your teen shows, the more you need to intervene—especially if he mentions or even thinks about suicide.

According to Dr. John Meeks, the following list of warning signs may indicate a possible teen suicide:

- Refuses to communicate with you
- Becomes more and more morose and isolated
- Shows a lack of enthusiasm for school—and a drop in grades
- Has recently become heavily involved with alcohol and drugs
- Is in the midst of family discord—arguments, tension, custody battles, and abuse
- Talks about a desire for revenge—against you
- Complains too much about aches and pains that have no physical basis
- Makes self-loathing comments
- Has little energy

- Has been recently rejected by a boyfriend or a girlfriend
- Has recently relocated to a new town or neighborhood
- Is living with a depressed parent or parents
- Has recently suffered the loss of a parent—from death, divorce, or separation
- Has overwhelming feelings of sadness and guilt
- Has frequent crying jags
- Acts overly nervous and withdrawn
- Is displaying slow speech and action
- Has been sleeping badly—either too much or too little
- Suffers from a learning disability that has been misdiagnosed for years
- Exhibits conduct disorder behavior—aggression, risk-taking, and antisocial acting out.
- Displays a morbid, obsessive fascination with death, dying, or violence—in movies, on TV, and in real life
- Has lost or gained too much weight too fast
- Feels hopeless and helpless about the future
- Has stopped seeing any friends—and has become more and more isolated
- Was close to someone who committed suicide
- Has given away a prized possession—a rare but "red flag" action
- Talks about suicide and death

THE UNIQUE CHARACTERISTICS OF SUICIDE

Approximately 500,000 teenagers every year try to kill themselves—and 5,500 of them succeed. But these figures might only be the tip of the iceberg. Some experts believe that the number of teens who commit suicide is really four times higher than these figures. Teenage suicide is a fact of life in today's world—a reality that crosses all economic, racial, social, and geographical lines. It knows teens intimately from all walks of life—from adolescents with involved, supportive parents to those with parents who couldn't care less, from delinquent kids who roam the streets to kids who grew up with the best of everything. It is a battle cry from the depths of despair—regardless of who sounds its call. Dr. Karl Menninger called suicide "the wish to kill, the wish to be killed, and the wish to die."

I believe there is another component: the wish to be free of pain.

HIGH-RISK FACTORS FOR SUCCESSFUL TEENAGE SUICIDE

Studies have shown that almost every teen who tries to commit suicide will have one or more of the following in his background:

- A strong desire to commit suicide
- A high degree of hopelessness and depression
- A history of suicide in the family
- Previous suicide attempts
- Social isolation and the lack of a good support system
- A history of antisocial behavior
- A recent loss or separation, including death, divorce, a move, or a graduation
- Substance abuse

With help, a suicidal teen can discover that freedom. But it is not always easy to see the warning signs. Over 80 percent of those teens who kill themselves talk about it before they act. Unfortunately, as we have seen, adolescents address their fears indirectly. They won't come out and say, "Please help me." Instead, their actions, their behavior, and their feelings do the talking—and it's up to us, the parents and the educators, to recognize the silent plea. Observing the symptoms in suicidal teens is only half the battle. Teenage suicide, like adolescence itself, is a complicated caldron of psychological, social, biological, and cultural forces. To fully understand why some teens try to kill themselves and others don't, you must go below the surface symptoms and understand this simmering brew of forces that, in the words of Macbeth's three witches, is full of "toil and trouble." Only then can you truly hear your teen's painful call—and offer real help.

An anonymous teenager in a Performance Group audience wrote: "How could you help someone if you think they want to commit suicide? How could you tell?" The answer to these questions is in these dramatic forces. Let's go over them now:

THE GLOBAL NEIGHBORHOOD: CULTURAL FORCES

1. A Question of Gender

Girls attempt suicide more than boys—but when boys try, they usually succeed. Here's proof: Ninety percent of the suicide attempts made each year are committed by girls—but 70 percent of all successful suicides are boys. The difference lies in their personalities. As we have seen, girls discuss their problems more openly than boys. They are less likely to let their feelings bottle up, and their cries for help will be more open. Boys, on the other hand, act more and talk less. They suffer in silence. By the time they decide to kill themselves, their pressures have already mounted to insupportable levels. Their minds are made up. They have an air of finality. There simply is no other way out. Girls also have a different view of suicide. To them, it has a romantic mystique. Like Catherine Earnshaw pining away for Heathcliff, they flirt with suicide when they've been rejected by a friend. This rejection becomes all-encompassing; not only are they rejected by their friends, but by their parents. Ultimately, they begin to reject themselves. In fact, one of the leading causes of suicide in girls is teenage pregnancy—both the anticipated fear and the reality. Like Ellen in the case study, these girls have often been abandoned by the boy they loved. They are terrified to tell their parents—who might reject them as well. Ultimately, they feel they have nowhere to turn, nowhere to go. The thought of the responsibility of motherhood overwhelms them—and they resort to suicide.

Finally, there is the choice of weapons. Girls usually resort to more passive, feminine methods of suicide, such as swallowing too many pills or slashing their wrists. But, as Sandra Gardner wrote in the book *Teenage Suicide,* boys use "more masculine, or violent methods— shooting, stabbing, jumping, hanging. These have less chance of rescue." Unfortunately, equality between the sexes has had one tragic result: Girls are beginning to use these more masculine methods to attempt suicide—and the number of them who succeed is climbing.

2. Ethnic Ties

Suicide among white middle-class boys is on the rise—a possible combination of the demands placed on them to succeed and the ease with which they can get alcohol or drugs. In fact, in one suicide study, almost all of the white male victims were intoxicated at the time of death. On the other hand, studies have found that blacks will try to commit suicide more than any other racial group. They grow up with solid family traditions and community ties, but as they approach young adulthood things change. They are confronted with the pain of racism, the lack of good job opportunities. As these young blacks move further and further away from their roots, they lose the solid ties that may have been shielding them from harsh reality. Full of impotent anger, they may act out in self-destructive ways—including "accidental" risk taking, drug overdosing, and suicide. Hispanics, too, often come from close-knit families. Their suicide rate is lower than those of both Caucasian and black teens. Suicide is most prevalent in Native American culture. It is the leading cause of death among teenage boys—possibly because of the erosion of the Indian way of life and the lack of self-esteem they experience in white society.

3. East Side, West Side

Suicide is a taboo in American culture. On a positive note, this will inhibit many teens from attempting it. But this same taboo will stop parents from recognizing that their teen is in trouble, or that his one attempt may very well be followed by another. A study of 752 families with teens who had tried to commit suicide found that the mothers were unaware of how deeply their children felt about suicide—even after their child's first try.

In Japan, suicide has also risen—partly because it is *not* as taboo. Suicide is considered a way to save face in Japanese society and, although not encouraged, it is accepted within their social and religious framework. Other reasons for the high rate of suicide include:

- extreme competition among Japanese youths
- a steadfast class system
- a college system based on an entrance exam that a student must pass—or be forever destined to failure
- a strict family structure

4. Geography Lesson

Contrary to popular belief, wide open spaces do not always offer serenity. More teenagers commit suicide in the western states and in Alaska than in any other area of the country. Suicides, of course, do occur in metropolitan areas, the Midwest, and the South, but studies suggest that the social isolation and the easier access to guns put western teenagers at higher risk. Despite all these cultural facts and figures, studies that have analyzed the statistics of teenage suicide have not been able to piece together a definitive pattern. No matter what your roots or where you live, there are other factors that make a teenager want to die.

SOCIETY'S CHILD: SOCIAL FORCES

5. Born in America

We live in a world where one out of every ten teens contemplates suicide, where suicide is the third leading cause of death in high school, and where, in a recent survey by the National Association of Private Psychiatric Hospitals, one third of all the questioned adults personally knew a teenager who either attempted or actually committed suicide. In this same survey, three quarters of the adults also believed that today's teens face far more serious problems than they did when they were young. These are, in many ways, "the worst of times." Families are splintering apart. Headlines read like science-fiction make-believe. Assassinations in China. Nuclear leaks, ozone layer leaks, and oil leaks. The prevalence of AIDS. All these things bombard our youth at a rapid, fast-paced clip. Add the fact that teens are still developing, searching, and experimenting with their new sense of self, and it makes sense that the pressure can become too much. Teens can't say, "Stop the world, I want to get off!" They can't plan a weekend away in solitude. Instead, some of them will strive to compete, to be perfect in their imperfect world—a goal that sets them up to fail. These are the Type A teens I discussed earlier, the student council presidents, the straight "A" students, the ones who looked as if they didn't have a care in the world.

But this is often a façade. As an anonymous teen wrote on an index card during a Performance Group, "When I attempted suicide in sixth grade it didn't really matter to me that I was near death. Now I realize how stupid I was. I tried because I lost a contest and couldn't bear being considered a loser." This teenager is not alone. Only 4 percent of these Type A teens commit suicide, but 30 percent give it serious thought. Other teens will "give up" on society rather than compete. They turn to drugs, alcohol, and delinquency to escape their confusion and their pain. Unfortunately, their numbers are growing. Teenage drug and alcohol abuse and crime have steadily risen over the years. And with their rise also comes an increase in the teenage suicide statistics.

6. The Media Monster

Romance has always played a role in entertainment. From war to love, corporate games to faraway fantasy, romance is always present. Heroes stand up for their beliefs—and win—if not the battle, then always the war. Love plays for keeps and good people win the prize. Movies, television, and books can inspire the most jaded adult. Teenagers, with their intensity, their susceptibility, and their naïveté, are even more susceptible to what they read and see. Sometimes the media's influence is good, providing role models, moral lessons, courage, and hope. But sometimes the negative power of the media is underestimated. Although the way sex and violence on television affect our youth is still being debated, programs that deal with teenage suicide have been proven, by Drs. Madelyn S. Gould and David Shaffer, to set it in motion unintentionally. In 1986 they set out to study the effects of four fictional television movies on teenage suicide. The plots of these movies were:

1. Two high school boys make a suicide pact.
2. A seventeen-year-old boy commits suicide after several personal crises.
3. A teenager tries to stop his father from committing suicide.
4. A boy and a girl commit suicide together.

All the movies were presented in a responsible manner by the production companies. Educational messages appeared at the end of each broadcast; numbers of suicide hotlines were placed on the screen; teachers' guides and scripts were made available to schools across the country. Yet, despite these measures, the doctors discovered that in the two-week period following each of the broadcasts, both attempted and successful suicides in the greater New York area significantly increased.

7. Clusters

Suicide breeds imitation—and not just by watching television movie broadcasts:

• Between September 1986 and October 1988, fourteen teenagers committed suicide in Cobb County, Georgia—and nine hundred residents there attempt suicide every year.

- On February 4, 1984, a thirteen-year-old boy committed suicide in Westchester County, New York. Ten days later, another boy in the same area joined him. Two days later, yet another boy shot himself. By the end of three weeks, five boys in the same area had killed themselves.
- In 1987 Bergenfield, New Jersey, was the scene for four teenage suicides. Only six days later, four other teens had also committed suicide in a Chicago suburb.

These suicides are part of a phenomenon called clusters—where one suicide will trigger several others. The American Psychiatric Association reports that these "clusters" are on the increase. But the good news is that because they give "advance notice," they can be prevented more effectively than isolated cases—if community leaders, educators, and parents combine forces to give their teens support and information.

8. Drug Talk

Substance abuse by itself does not cause suicide. Rather, it is a vehicle that accelerates the pace. Teens who take drugs are more at risk, because they usually have low self-control, and stress affects them more easily. They also have a tendency to act impulsively when under the influence of either drugs or alcohol. And the drugs themselves make an easy and accessible weapon to end their lives.

Teenagers often take drugs to treat depression. But, ultimately, a teen will find that the drugs he is taking are making things not better but worse. And, when drugs fail, a teen is left with a tremendous sense of despair. He has lost not only his familiar "best friend," but also his only way of coping with stress. There's only one way out: suicide.

9. Risky Business

The Rebel-Without-a-Cause demeanor. Fast cars and motorcycles. Drinking while driving. Drag races and death-defying bets. This is the cliché of the self-proclaimed delinquent, the troubled adolescent hell-bent on destruction who, more times than not, ends up a suicide statistic. Risk-taking behavior may be a symptom of a wish to die.

Car accidents. Motorcycle crashes. Drug overdoses. Many of these "accidental" deaths are, in reality, disguised suicide attempts.

A BODY OF FACTS: BIOLOGICAL FORCES

10. A Chemistry Lesson

The body and the mind work together. Teenage suicide is as much a product of biology as of emotions. As with depression, a chemical imbalance in the brain can actually promote suicidal thoughts and actions. In chapter seven, we have seen how an imbalance of serotonin, a neurotransmitter that carries messages to various parts of the brain, promotes poor impulse control and aggression in conduct-disordered teens. Low levels of serotonin have also been found in suicidal people. Studies have found that people who took their lives in violent ways—from shooting to jumping to hanging—had extremely low levels of serotonin. Growth hormone secretions have also been found to influence teenage suicide. A study of 140 adolescents between the ages of twelve and eighteen found that thirty-four of them had growth hormone deficiencies in their brains. These same thirty-four teens were severely depressed and had also attempted suicide.

THE INNER BURDEN: PSYCHOLOGICAL FORCES

11. A View of Death

Teenagers see life and death through different eyes than adults. Recognizing this difference is crucial for successful suicide prevention in adolescents. Understanding the concept of death and mortality is a process that comes only with age:

- To an infant there is no such thing as death. Before the age of one, children cannot comprehend that death exists at all.
- Between the ages of one and five, children perceive death as a changeable occurrence. To them, death is a temporary intrusion that can be changed by choice.
- From five to nine death becomes much more intimate for children. They see it as magical and frightening—something from the far-off reaches of a dark fantasy land.
- When children reach the age of nine they begin to develop an understanding of what death truly is. But, through the teenage years and beyond, they see death as a far-off event—it is of no immediate interest to them.

Suicidal thoughts are also a product of age. Suicide is seldom seen in children under twelve. Some studies suggest that this is because their concept of death is not mature. Other research claims they haven't developed enough cognitive skills to plan a successful strategy for suicide. Still other studies have found that feelings of hopelessness, the despair that leads to suicide, are not in place until the onset of puberty. But even with their cognitive skills, their festering despair, and their more mature concept of mortality, adolescents still do not see the finality of death. They see themselves going toward a better life—or believe they can come back as a better person. As a teenager in the Performance Group said, "I didn't think of death as final. I thought I'd die and come back and everything would be fine. I wouldn't be a drug addict anymore."

Teenagers who attempt suicide see it as a solution, not a problem. They do not want death; they want relief. In fact, 70 percent of all teenage suicide attempts occur between three P.M. and twelve midnight—when someone will be home.

THE BORDERLINE STORY

Only 8 to 10 percent of people suffering from borderline personality disorders actually commit suicide, but many of them do threaten suicide to manipulate those around them and get what they want. Often the result of an impaired separation and individuation development, borderline personality disorders are rarely found in adolescents, but even one is too many. Here, according to the DSM-III-R, are its symptoms:

- A pattern of unstable and intense interpersonal relationships
- Impulsive, self-damaging behavior—including shoplifting, binge eating, promiscuous sex, spending, reckless driving, and substance abuse
- Extreme mood swings—from depression to anxiety
- Inappropriate anger—or lack of anger
- Recurrent suicidal threats
- Disturbed and uncertain self-identity—including body image, sexual orientation, goals, types of friends, and values
- Chronic boredom and emptiness
- Frantic efforts to avoid real or imagined abandonment

When adolescents swallow too many aspirins, they aren't thinking of that "black void," that place of no return. Instead, they might be:

1. Trying to punish a parent or a rejecting friend: "They'll be sorry they hurt me!" One study of teenage suicide found that half the notes left by suicide victims contained hostility directed at other people or events.
2. Directing that anger at themselves, needing to inflict self-punishment for real or imagined "crimes"—though only two of the suicide victims in the study noted above left notes with self-loathing comments.
3. Imitating their parents—who have suicidal tendencies themselves.
4. Wishing to "join" a beloved relative or friend who recently died.

12. Family Feeling

As you might expect, the psychological and social environment of the family combined with the medical and mental history of family members can significantly influence a suicidal teen. Lack of family communication, family hostility and depression, family fights, divorce, and discord can leave a teen feeling isolated and unloved—and susceptible to suicide.

Most experts agree: The home environment is a critical factor in every adolescent disorder, including suicidal tendencies. A suicide in the family increases the risk six times for teens.

Here are some other family factors:

A depressed parent breeds discontent and is a negative role model. In the same way nurturing, positive messages are passed from parent to child, so is self-destructive behavior. A study comparing the parents of forty-six teenage suicide attempters with the parents of forty-six nonsuicidal teenagers found more depression, more alcohol consumption, and lower self-esteem in the fathers of the suicide attempters. Their mothers also drank more than the mothers of nonsuicidal teens and were more anxious and suicidal themselves.

Sexual and physical abuse can lead to suicide attempts. Studies have discovered that children who have been abused blame themselves and consider themselves wicked. This feeling of self-loathing makes them highly susceptible to suicide.

A lack of communication in families can be deadly. As we have seen, families are resistant to change. They prefer to sweep problems away instead of admitting that their teen is in trouble—and that the family equilibrium might be disrupted forever.

Sometimes this lack of communication stems from insecurity. Emotionally needy parents can't meet their own needs, let alone those of their child. These parents want their child to tell them they are indeed good parents. They don't want to hear about the confusion their teen might be feeling or about his latest problem in school. Instead, they convey the message, "Just the good news, please." Unfortunately, their children learn not to communicate—which spreads to their friends and their teachers. They become more and more isolated, more and more troubled.

Sometimes talk just isn't a family's way. Many parents feel that communication means giving orders to their teen. It's "Sit down and eat your breakfast" or "Go on upstairs and do your homework." Dr. Vincent Fontana, head of the New York City Task Force on Child Abuse, calls this family atmosphere an "emotional refrigerator," and one that fosters suicidal tendencies in teens.

Family discord can also be a factor. In fact, almost three quarters of all teenage suicide attempters report family problems—including lack of support and instability. When stress and conflict are a way of life, there is no security. Without security there can be no trust. A child who can't trust his parents will feel helpless and vulnerable. He might fear his parents' discipline. He might feel guilty, believing he caused their distress. He might feel angry at them for fighting, which only compounds his guilt. To escape his intolerable home and his intolerable feelings, he might see only one way out: suicide.

13. High Anxiety

Teens are impulsive, and they will plunge into things without considering the long-term consequences. When a teen is troubled, this impulsive streak can become deadly. All that's needed is a stressful life event to put a teenager "over the edge," to make her leap into suicide without looking.

Studies have found that anxiety is a strong predictor of short-term suicidal behavior—the type of suicidal feelings that occur after a stressful life event. The less a teen can cope with stress, the more anxiety she will feel. The more anxiety she feels, the more she might impulsively seek out suicide after a traumatic event. And what teens call a traumatic event might be considered trivial by adults. A teenage suicide can be triggered by such seemingly mundane events as a failing grade or a snub at school. In fact, the most common situation that puts a teen "over the edge" involves punishment. Anticipating parental or legal discipline, whether for cutting school or smashing up the car, has often been found to trigger suicide. Some triggering traumas, however, aren't "trivial" at all. The death of a parent. A custody battle. A divorce. Eighty percent of suicidal teens have lost a parent in one of these ways before they were fourteen.

14. The First Semester

Higher learning can breed higher anxiety. Here are some cruel, hard facts:

- Suicide is the leading cause of death among college students.
- Every year ten thousand college students try to kill themselves— and between five hundred and one thousand succeed. College life brings its own brand of stress. Not only are incoming students still experiencing the normal adolescent conflicts of high-school days, but they are experiencing them in a whole new environment. Culture shock. Fierce competition. Homesickness. Career anxiety. Loneliness. Academic and collegiate pressures. Any or all of these elements can make a teenager depressed enough to think of suicide.

15. The Inside Story

We do live in turbulent times. Some theories of suicide suggest that the feelings of hopelessness combined with the tenuousness of a world dominated by the threat of nuclear war, and widespread starvation and homelessness, may be major factors in the rise in teen suicide since the 1950s. I disagree. Suicidal thoughts originate inside the teenager, not with current events. The battle lines that determine a potentially suicidal teen are drawn between conflicting psychological and social pressures.

As we have seen earlier, most teenagers develop in positive ways. They are proud of their new bodies and have a healthy self-identity. They are excited and enthusiastic about their futures. But some teens get stuck in the developmental process. Instead of celebrating their new beginnings, they mourn their loss—of childhood, of heroic parental figures, of an innocence that never really existed. The reasons are many: a dysfunctional family, a problem in the separation and individuation process, learning impairment, an inability to cope with stressful life events. Unfortunately, teens don't recognize that they are mourning. Instead, they become depressed. Self-doubt and insecurity roam free, posing questions without end: Do my friends like me? Will my father die? How can I go outside with a body like this? Will I get into college? Why can't I be normal? These teens will begin to hate themselves. Their search for self-identity often ends in self-loathing. They become afraid to talk. To communicate what they are going through means setting themselves up for rejection or ridicule from family and friends. They're not even sure what exactly they are feeling. All they know is that they feel helpless, hopeless, and unloved.

It's a vicious cycle. The more helpless and hopeless a teen feels, the less she will want to talk about it. The less she talks about it, the greater her feelings of despair and isolation. A study of suicidal teens by Dr. Michael L. Peck and Dr. Robert E. Litman found that their feelings sprang from not being understood or appreciated by their parents and an inability to express themselves. Ninety percent of these same teens didn't feel their parents understood them at all.

Family, friends, school, and adolescence itself all require strong coping skills. If a teen has not learned how to deal with his conflicting emotions, his pain, and the daily stresses of teenage life, he can lose the inner battle—and lose his life.

Treating Suicide

Attempted suicide is an emergency situation. Sometimes hospitalization is required to bring a child back to physical health. But even after the crisis has passed, it still waits to loom again—in the form of another attempt. Physical health is only part of the story—even if a teen promises never to try suicide again. Attempts usually beget subsequent attempts—unless the underlying depression, the dysfunctional family, the inability to cope with life's stress are treated.

The best place for treatment is a hospital. Away from the environment that set them off teens can build up their confidence and their self-esteem. They can learn better coping skills. They can gain insight on their problems and their family's problems that will enable them to accept their lives and move on. Medications can also be closely monitored and adjusted as the need arises.

Prevention is the key to all adolescent disorders—but nowhere is it more important than with teenage suicide. Here there is not always a second chance. A teenager who is thinking about suicide must be helped before she puts her thoughts into action. A teenager who has tried to kill herself must be stopped from trying again.

Preventing the tragedy of teenage suicide can be a reality. But we must recognize our youths' cry for help. We must implement programs within the community to educate and support both parents and teens. And we must fight our own fears, our own taboos about suicide, so the helpful advice we give rings true. As the teenagers in the Performance Group sing:

We have to stick together
We need some help from one another.
It's up to me and you to see this through.
It's up to me and you to see this through.

We have now gone over the most common adolescent disorders. We have heard our children's ultimate cry for help. It's now time to turn to the various treatments available in today's world, from medicines for the mind to individual, group, and family therapies. It is time to move on to the treatment, to the happy ending that is not only a possibility, but a proven fact for both teenagers and their parents everywhere.

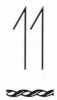

MEDICATIONS

Linda had been an "A" student until her family moved to a different state. During the first five months in her new school, Linda's grades dropped to "D's" and "F's." She went to her room and stayed there as soon as she got home from school. She stopped eating and she refused to talk to anyone. Her parents brought her to an adolescent psychiatrist who put her on nortriptyline, an antidepressant. Within four weeks, her depression lifted. Today, she continues to take her medication in conjunction with biweekly therapy.

Jimmy had always suffered from extreme mood swings. One week he'd be enthusiastic, exuberant, and confident; the next he'd be in the throes of a deep depression. Because he was a good student and had several close friends, his parents assumed he was acting like a typical teen. But in the month before he was to start college, he hit rock bottom. He tried to kill himself. Jimmy's parents brought him to a hospital with an adolescent unit. He was put on lithium, which alleviated his terrible low states and kept his highs in balance.

Denise had been diagnosed as bulimic over two years ago. Although she had been in both individual and group therapy since that time, she continued to binge and purge herself every few weeks. She said she wasn't depressed or upset about anything in her life; she simply couldn't help herself. Her parents didn't know what to do; they were almost at the end of their rope. They brought her to Fair Oaks Hospital where she was put on imipramine, a medication normally used for depression. Within six weeks, Linda's bulimic cycle stopped completely.

Carson had always had a problem with attention. When he was in grade school, he was unruly and hyperactive. His parents had him tested at that time and the results showed no physical problems. They were told that he was simply "more active than other kids his age." But Carson's misconduct continued when he entered seventh grade. His grades were bad; he had few friends. He began to act out in more dangerous ways than simply talking back to a teacher. When he vandalized the school cafeteria, his parents brought him to an adolescent psychiatrist. Carson was put on Ritalin, a stimulant, which helped his attention span. Because he could now sit still and pay attention for longer periods of time, his hyperactive behavior stopped. He is about to graduate high school with honors this June.

These teens are not alone. They are among the millions of adolescents who have benefited from the new medicines of the mind, the strange-sounding drugs that read more like "Jeopardy" stumpers than forms of therapeutic treatment.

A mere forty years ago, these drugs were unknown. Depressions and other psychological disorders were considered illnesses of the mind that had nothing to do with the body. People who were depressed or anxious were called hysterical or worse. Today we understand the vital link between the mind and the body in ways that Freud or his colleagues never could have imagined. We know that psychological disorders are very much rooted in biology—and that brain matter itself can dictate our emotions, thoughts, and behaviors. In the same way our arterial system can start a coronary heart attack in motion, a malfunctioning brain can create psychological pain.

MATTER OVER MIND

Biopsychiatry and psychopharmacology are the medical bywords for the nineties. Thanks to these two sciences our views on depression, anxiety, and irrationality have been forever changed. Because of biopsychiatry, we have made tremendous advances in our knowledge of neurotransmitters, the chemical impulses that carry messages throughout the brain. This science has also taught us much more about specific brain sections, those separate gray areas that carry out the tasks the neurotransmitters' messages have relayed. At the same time, psychopharmacology has enabled us to better understand the effects of mood-altering drugs, creating safer, more predictable, and more effective medicines of the mind. Combined with the appropriate psychotherapy, these two fields have brought us new hope and new success in treating psychological disorders—in both adults and adolescents alike.

But scientific inroads are not enough. Even though we have entered the last decade of the twentieth century, we have still held on to the misconceptions, the misinformation, and the myths of the past—including our erroneous beliefs about pharmaceutical drugs. Many people today are still afraid of these mood-altering medications. Like those who sneer at anything newfangled, many people don't trust these new drugs. Before drugs can be administered successfully, the air must be cleared and destructive medication myths must be dispelled. To help demystify the medication your teen might have to take, here are some common myths people have about today's psychiatric drugs, along with the proven facts:

MYTH: These psychiatric medications are not safe for growing adolescents.

FACT: When they are administered by a competent and experienced physician, these medicines are extremely safe—as long as your teen follows doctor's instructions.

MYTH: If a teenager gets depressed, all he has to do is talk to somebody. He'll get over it with time.

FACT: As we have seen in previous chapters, clinical depression and other psychological disorders will only get worse if they are not treated. Because many disorders are a result of a chemical imbalance in the brain, medication is usually needed in conjunction with other therapy. An antidepressant can stave off a depression's more severe symptoms— and give the insights learned in psychotherapy or skill training a chance to "sink in." A stimulant can keep hyperactivity at bay and give school instructions and remedial education skills a chance to do their job. An antianxiety medication can calm a teen down and give him a chance to work on his separation and individuation problems unencumbered by excess fear. Approximately 70 percent of all troubled persons are helped with a combination of medication and other forms of therapy.

MYTH: All antidepressants are the same.

FACT: Many antidepressant medications are similar. But, as with antibiotics, for example, individuals may respond differently to different drugs. One depressed teen might do well with imipramine. Another might do better with nortriptyline. A teenager's age, personal habits, physical health, and metabolism all help a doctor determine which drug to give, what dosage to recommend, how long it should be taken, and how well it works. Further, he or she might choose one medication over another based on a particular drug's success rate and the severity of its side effects. A good physician will always try to match the right drug with the right patient, as well as supervise and check its dosage, reactions, and levels in the blood during the entire drug therapy process to ensure the medication's continued effectiveness.

MYTH: Psychiatric medications are just another way for a teen to get high.

FACT: Contrary to popular opinion, psychiatric medications do not provide a high in depressed people, but simply help them return to a more normal and balanced emotional state. And the medications have no psychological effect in people who are not biologically depressed. To illuminate this point, think of these medications as aspirin. If you have a high fever, the aspirin will bring it down. But if your temperature is normal, aspirin will have no effect. There is one crucial factor regarding these medications that every parent must understand: Although they are not abused by teens, *antidepressants are the number-one drug used in teenage suicides.* They do take time to work and require some patience—something an adolescent has in short supply. A teenager who is already severely depressed might reach for his pills to harm himself. It is therefore imperative for parents to monitor the daily administration of the antidepressants—until they've at least had a chance to take effect. For suicidal teens, short-term hospitalization might be recommended so that medications can be closely supervised twenty-four hours a day.

MYTH: Psychiatric drugs are overprescribed.

FACT: Unfortunately, medicines of the mind are usually underprescribed—thanks to preconceived notions and misguided information. These medications are also not always given in strong enough amounts to teens. Studies have found that teenagers require higher doses of antidepressants than their adult counterparts—possibly because the most developmental changes in neurotransmitter structures occur during adolescence. Unfortunately, a lower dosage can translate into a lower level of therapeutic benefit. Because they are not getting the medication they need, many teens don't show any improvement. Both they and their parents get discouraged and stop the drug treatment, when, in actuality, the medicine can be effective. The teen simply needs a higher dose.

DR. NO'S

The best medicine in the world can't work if a teenager uses caffeine, alcohol, or nicotine. If your teen drinks a lot of coffee or if he is smoking, it's important your doctor know. Both caffeine and nicotine can decrease a drug's effectiveness. Neither of these two "drugs" negative effects come close to alcohol. The combination of psychiatric drugs and alcohol can, at best, neutralize the drug's benefits. At worst, the results can be deadly.

MYTH: Medication will inhibit a teenager's moral, cognitive, and physical growth.

FACT: Although there has been much more research on adult versus adolescent psychopharmacology, no study has been able to prove that taking medications will physically or psychologically harm a teenager. They can only help him. Stimulants, for example, can help a teenager curb his problems with impulse control. The more control he has over his hyperactivity, the more he can learn what is socially appropriate. And the more he is able to control his impulses, the more readily he will learn moral responsibility. A teenager involved in a complete treatment program receives the chance to understand what his problems are and how to cope with them. He can end up light-years ahead of other kids his age who have not had the same opportunity to gain insight into their behavior. As the saying goes, "No pain, no gain."

MYTH: Drug therapy is the answer to every teenage disorder.

FACT: These medications are not magic. They are not a cure-all for problems that will always arise in life. They must always be combined with other forms of therapy, and they must always be used under a doctor's close supervision. Ultimately, a teenager must learn better ways to cope with life's traumas. She must accept who she is. She must find positive ways to grow. None of these things can be found from swallowing a pill. They require insight and problem-solving skills— qualities that can come only from a variety of therapy programs.

A DOCTOR'S COMPLIANCE CHECKLIST

Some of the questions doctors consider to determine whether their patients will stick with a drug treatment program:

- Is there a history of noncompliance?
- Are there family problems at home that might interfere with the patient's compliance?
- What is the patient's tolerance for side effects?
- Is the dosage schedule too complex to follow easily?
- Do the patient and his family accept responsibility for taking the drug?
- Does the patient completely understand the instructions for taking the medication?
- Does the patient keep scheduled therapy appointments?
- Can the patient's family afford the drugs?
- Is there a good, supportive relationship between the patient and the therapist?

Reprinted with minor changes from *Aftershock: Surviving the Delayed Effects of Trauma, Crisis and Loss* by Andrew E. Slaby, M.D., Ph.D. (New York: Villard Books, 1989).

ENEMY INFILTRATION

Throughout this book, we have seen how teenagers are different from adults. When it comes to medication, there is one way in which they are the same. Teenagers, like their adult counterparts, can hinder a drug's effectiveness through noncompliance. This is not medical terminology for ignoring a parent. Nor does it have anything to do with punishment. In general terms, noncompliance means a failure to comply with someone or something. In the medical world, it means a patient's failure to take his or her medication. There are many reasons why both adults and teens suffer from noncompliance. For teens all these reasons are complicated by the fact that their parents are also involved. Teenagers need their parents' help, especially if they are severely depressed and in danger of committing suicide. As Dr. Laurence L. Greenhill states in *The Clinical Guide to Child Psychiatry,* "The parents form the key to success in the treatment of the child with psychoactive drugs." Instead of one variable, there are two. Parents can decide their teen is healthy—and doesn't need to take medicine anymore. Because medication takes several weeks to take effect, parents can decide it isn't working and discontinue treatment. Or they can grow tired of constantly supervising their teen and forget to administer a pill once in a while. Teens, too, can decide the pills aren't working and not take the prescribed dosage. They can become tired of being treated like children by their parents and refuse to take their medication. And at a time when acceptance is so important, they can feel like outsiders—forced to be different because they have to take a pill during lunch or when they're out on a date. A teen can also consider the medicine as punishment instead of treatment. Here's an example:

For several months, Jimmy has had violent fits of temper, breaking lamps and ashtrays, and hurling pillows across the room. His parents, of course, were very upset, and they were pleased that the stimulants Jimmy began taking stopped his dangerous tantrums. But Jimmy feels that his parents caused him to get angry in the first place. He sees the medicine he has to take as punishment and something he doesn't really need. Further, he views his therapist as an enemy in cahoots with his parents. But Jimmy will show them all: He'll simply stop taking his medication.

As this anecdote illuminates, it is crucial that both you and your teen have a dialogue with the psychiatrist administering the psychiatric drug. Drugs are a complicated issue. They do take time to work. They can induce certain initial side effects—dizziness, nausea, or drowsiness—which, if a family is unprepared, can create fear and promote further noncompliance. When it comes to successful drug therapy, both you and your child must understand what it is, how it works—and why.

Parents can also provide positive support. Unlike a single, isolated adult, a teenager does have a network of people to keep noncompliance at bay. Here, from *When Acting Out Isn't Acting* by Drs. Lynne W. Weisberg and Rosalie Greenberg, is a short "wrong" and "right" dialogue that shows how parents can help their teen stay with their medication:

WRONG: Boy, those pills really work. Your grades have gotten so much better since you started taking them.

RIGHT: Your grades are much better now. Those pills let you show how smart you really are.

PILL TALK

Like any other science, psychopharmacology and biopsychiatry are not exact. As Dr. Andrew E. Slaby puts it in his book *Aftershock:* "Mathematics solves one equation only to find infinite possibilities in its answer. Astronomy discovers one star only to find an entire galaxy behind it. Medicine heralds one breakthrough cure only to find it can be improved. The possibilities are always there." Even as I write this, progress is being made in pharmaceuticals, creating new variables and new discoveries. But, in general, the following statements hold true:

- *Depression* is usually treated with antidepressants or mood-stabilizing medications such as lithium.
- *Aggressive disorders* are usually treated with stimulants or antidepressants.
- *Anxiety disorders* are usually treated with antidepressants, minor tranquilizers and/or antiobsessive medication.
- *Personality disorders* are usually treated with antidepressants, lithium, or major tranquilizers (also called antipsychotics).

As you can see, different disorders require different medications—or sometimes a combination of two or more. To help you recognize the wide variety of available drugs, I've compiled a short descriptive list of the more common ones. It is my hope that this information will cut through some of the confusion in today's "medicine show," and that it will help you gain insight into and understanding of a form of therapy that is changing the theater of the mind for good.

NOTE: **Remember that NONE of this material can take the place of a doctor's knowledge or experience. And no drug should be given without a doctor's supervision.**

Antidepressants

The good news is that antidepressants work in 60 to 85 percent of all diagnosed depressions. The bad news is that they take several weeks to take effect. They can also have uncomfortable side effects. Even though these are short-lived, some patients might not be able to tolerate them.

Tricyclic Antidepressants (TCAs)
Use: Depression disorders. Underlying depressions in various other illnesses, including eating disorders, anxiety disorders, and conduct

disorders. May be used in attention-deficit hyperactivity disorders when stimulants do not work.

OBSESSIVE-COMPULSIVE DISORDER: THE DRUG OF CHOICE

Between one third and one half of all obsessive-compulsive disorders (OCD) begin in childhood and adolescence. Treating the disorder during these developmental years can prevent problems in adulthood. One medication, a new TCA antidepressant called clomipramine, has had startlingly good results in adolescents with obsessive-compulsive disorder. In a five-week study of twenty-one adolescents with OCD, clomipramine was found to be far superior than a more common antidepressant in treating the disorder. Though widely used in Europe and in Canada, clomipramine is currently available in the United States only on a "compassionate use" basis. (Parents of OCD children should ask their physician about this medication.)

Characteristics: So named because of their three-ring molecular structure, TCAs help stabilize the level of the brain's chemical neurotransmitters. They also appear to prevent catecholamine levels (a stimulating chemical in the brain sometimes referred to as neurotransmitters) from increasing (see chapter nine).

The TCAs most commonly prescribed for adolescents are nortriptyline and imipramine. A study of two groups of school phobics, one who took imipramine and one who took a placebo (a "fake" pill that the group thought was real), found that the imipramine was highly effective. In the placebo-taking group, only 47 percent returned to school—and only 21 percent felt better. But among the group that took imipramine, 81 percent returned to school and 100 percent felt better.

Some common brand names: Elavil, Pamelor, Norpramin, and Tofranil.

Possible side effects: Blurry vision, constipation, dry mouth, rapid pulse, sleepiness, difficult urination.

Withdrawal: Gradual reduction under a doctor's supervision.

MAO Inhibitors
Use: An older medication, these antidepressants are used when TCAs don't work or sometimes in combination with a TCA under a doctor's strict supervision.

Characteristics: During adolescence, estrogen production is at its highest, which can prevent a TCA from doing its job. MAO inhibitors work differently. They block a malfunctioning enzyme called monamine oxidase (MAO) from breaking down the chemical neurotransmitters in the brain and causing depression. They have also been proven more effective in depressions where too much sleep and overeating are factors.

MAOs must be strictly supervised. All fermented foods such as beer, cheese, and wine must be completely avoided—as well as over-the-counter medications for hay fever, coughs, and colds. The combination of the two can be fatal, resulting in extreme high blood pressure and possible death. Because teenagers are notorious for their cavalier diets, TCAs are always tried first. But if your teen needs to take an MAO inhibitor, this dietary rule must be brought home. Ask your doctor or pharmacist for a complete list of those foods and medications that must be avoided.

Some common brand names: Nardil, Marplan, and Parnate.

Possible side effects: Headaches, high blood pressure, irregular pulse, nausea, vomiting, light sensitivity, and stiff neck.

Withdrawal: Gradual tapering off under a doctor's supervision.

Mood Stabilizers

Manic depression is usually seen in adults. But more and more cases have been discovered in a person's late teens and early twenties. As we have seen in chapter four, the earlier a manic depression (or bipolar depression) is caught and treated, the less havoc it will create in a teenager's ongoing development.

Lithium Carbonate
Use: In manic-depressive disorders. Lithium has also been used successfully with oversocialized, aggressive conduct disorders and in teens with ADHD who don't respond well to stimulants.

Characteristics: A natural mineral salt, lithium has been found to prevent manic episodes in 70 percent of all cases—as well as to soften the extreme intensity of the depressive cycles.

Because lithium reacts with fluids (called electrolytes) that have been chemically broken down in the body, a teenager who exercises strenuously in the heat, who perspires excessively, who is on a salt or liquid restrictive diet, or who is currently taking diuretics must be closely monitored.

Some common brand names: Lithane, Lithobid, and Eskalith.

Possible side effects: Confusion, tremor, sleepiness, headaches, diarrhea, nausea, rashes, restlessness, and hallucinations. These are usually dose-related.

Withdrawal: Many doctors recommend that lithium be continued at least one year after adolescence. At that time, a drug "vacation" can be taken to see how the young adult copes without medication.

Carbamazepine

Use: When lithium doesn't work—or in combination with it.

Characteristics: Similar in chemical structure to the antidepressant imipramine, carbamazepine was previously used only to prevent convulsions in epilepsy disorders. Today, it has proven a successful medication in 50 percent of bipolar disorders. Because its side effects can be extremely dangerous, it must be used only with a doctor's strict supervision—and only when lithium alone has failed.

Common brand name: Tegretol.

Possible Side effects: Drowsiness, irritability, and a possible suppression of blood-cell production. Before prescribing this medication, a physician must perform a complete physical exam that includes a blood-cell work-up.

Withdrawal: Gradual reduction under a doctor's supervision.

Stimulants

The pros and cons of stimulants have been debated everywhere—from the most rarefied professional scientific journals to the most widely syndicated television talk shows. But the fact always remains that they work—in 80 percent of all hyperactive cases.

People have long believed that stimulants have an opposite effect in children than they do in adults. Instead of making them more "hyper," stimulants make children calm. However, scientists now know this "paradoxical effect" is not what happens at all. Stimulants don't attack a teen's hyperactivity. But they do work on his attention span. By becoming more focused, a teen will automatically become less hyper. Paying attention means paying attention—not running around the room or drawing on the cafeteria wall. Stimulants have also been found to stop antisocial behavior in teens and in adults as well.

A correct dosage is paramount. Too much and a child can become a zombie. Too little and there will be no change in behavior. Some studies of stimulants have discovered slight cognitive and growth impairment, while others have indicated absolutely no impairment. The benefits gained from properly supervised stimulants—less disruptive, aggressive behavior, better school performance, better disposition and social skills, even improved athletic performance—far outweigh any unproven negatives. Effective stimulant treatment has even been found to decrease the risk of alcohol and drug abuse in later life. If a teen turns out to be unresponsive or dysfunctional from stimulant medication, there are other forms of treatment, including antidepressants, which your physician can try.

Methylphenidate
Use: In teens diagnosed with ADHD and conduct disorders.

Characteristics: This stimulant appears to work on the catecholamine in the brain to increase impulse control and concentration. Studies have found that both young children and adolescents can benefit from this drug—but it is most effective when given several times a day instead of in a time-release form. Unfortunately, having to take pills frequently can promote noncompliance, especially among peer-conscious teens.

Common brand name: Ritalin.

Possible side effects: Headache, rapid heartbeat, stomachache, dizziness, changes in blood pressure, initial insomnia, weight loss, or continued irritability and hyperactivity. Teenagers who have a family history of Tourette's syndrome or tic disorder should not take Ritalin.

Withdrawal: Ritalin is recommended throughout adolescence—with regular drug vacations to determine if the stimulant treatment is still needed.

Dextroamphetamine sulfate
Use: In cases where Ritalin does not work.

Characteristics: This stimulant is older than Ritalin and is available in more varieties, including liquid, slow-release capsules, and tablets. It is a controlled substance that must be given more than once a day for optimum benefit.

Common brand name: Dexedrine.

Possible side effects: Headache, dizziness, stomachache, rapid heartbeat, changes in blood pressure, appetite suppression.

Withdrawal: Dexedrine can be given throughout adolescence—with periodic drug vacations to determine if it is still needed.

Magnesium Pemoline.
Use: In cases where the side effects of both Dexedrine and Ritalin prove insurmountable and in teens who have difficulty taking medications during the school day.

SURVIVING ADOLESCENCE 181

Characteristics: This medication is fairly new. Because its effects are longer-lasting, a single dose a day can do the job. However, it does take three weeks to "kick in"—and both teens and parents must be patient.

Common brand name: Cylert.

Possible side effects: Dizziness, headaches, stomachaches, rapid heartbeat, changes in blood pressure, and possible liver abnormalities. Occasional liver function tests must be administered by your physician.

Withdrawal: Cylert treatment can continue throughout your teen's adolescent years. Occasional drug vacations can help determine if the dosage should be changed or if it can be discontinued.

Antianxiety Drugs

Antianxiety medications include the benzodiazepines—the most widely prescribed psychiatric medications for adults. But adolescents are different, and the possibility of substance abuse is always a critical consideration when prescribing these medications to teens. Physicians will usually try an antidepressant first, especially because TCAs have had success in treating phobias and anxiety states. But if an anxiety-disordered teen does not respond to the antidepressant, or if the teen suffers from chronic anxiety, a benzodiazepine may be administered with careful supervision.

Benzodiazepines (BZs)

Use: Treatment of anxiety disorders, including panic attacks, phobias, and obsessive-compulsive behavior.

Characteristics: The BZs inhibit central nervous system excitement by acting on its benzodiazepine nerve endings. They do their work before an anxiety attack begins, stopping the fearful anticipation of a situation rather than halting it midstream. Alcohol must always be avoided when BZs are taken and, because of their potential for abuse, BZs are usually given only for short periods of time. They treat symptoms but not the actual disease; the reasons for a teenager's anxiety must be explored with other forms of therapy.

Some common brand names: Valium, Xanax, Librium, and Ativan.

Possible side effects: Drowsiness, fatigue, mild depression, dry mouth, and temporary confusion and loss of motor coordination.

Withdrawal: BZs must be gradually discontinued. Abrupt withdrawal can result in extreme anxiety and convulsions.

Another mild tranquilizer, **buspirone,** is currently being used under the brand name BuSpar. Although it has the same calming effects of

BZs, BuSpar is not a benzodiazepine, and initial studies have indicated that it may not be as potentially habit-forming as other antianxiety medications.

Antihistamines
Use: Treating anxiety—especially when it creates psychosomatic cold-like symptoms.

Characteristics: Creates a general calming effect. Because they are not as habit-forming as BZs, antihistamines might be tried first for teens suffering from anxiety disorders.

Some common brand names: Atarax, Benadryl, and Vistaril.

Possible side effects: Drowsiness, fatigue, dry mouth, and possible hyperactivity (especially in teens suffering from a concurrent conduct disorder). Alcohol will intensify any drowsiness and should be avoided.

Withdrawal: Medication should be gradually discontinued to avoid the return of an anxious state.

Beta Blockers (BBs)
Use: Treating anxiety, especially stage fright.

Characteristics: Although these common heart medications are not literally a minor tranquilizer, BBs can alleviate anticipated tension and fear. But instead of acting on the central nervous system, this medication works on the peripheral nervous system—blocking a teen's automatic responses to outside stimuli. Rapid heartbeat, elevated blood pressure, hyperventilation: All these physical symptoms of anxiety are stopped before they can occur. And, by reducing these symptoms, anxiety is also lowered.

Some common brand names: Inderal, Tenormin, Corgard, Lopressor.

Possible side effects: Insomnia, asthma, nausea, and fatigue.

Withdrawal: This medication should be gradually reduced under a doctor's supervision.

Antipsychotics or Major Tranquilizers

These drugs are as serious as they sound. Sometimes called neuroleptics, sometimes called major tranquilizers, and sometimes called antipsychotics, they are used for severely troubled teens. These medications work on the chemical imbalance of dopamine and serotonin in the brain, regulating emotions and producing a sense of calm.

Because adolescent psychoses such as schizophrenia do not show the same delusions, hallucinations, or strange thoughts and behaviors of its adult counterparts, major tranquilizers are less effective on teens. However, they do serve a purpose in curbing agitation, hyperactivity, and extreme aggression.

Phenothiazines
Use: This medication is primarily used in treating severe brain damage, schizophrenia, and autism. It is also used for psychotic episodes of extreme aggression and hyperactivity.

Characteristics: Research has shown that phenothiazines are effective in treating adolescent schizophrenia. However, various studies have not been able to prove their effectiveness in treating nonpsychotic adolescents who might be suffering from overanxiety or aggression. Because of the possibility of developing tardive dyskinesia, a condition characterized by sudden facial tics or body jerkiness, they are considered drugs of last resort.

Some common brand names: Thorazine, Trilafon, Stelazine, Prolixin, and Mellaril.

Possible side effects: Drowsiness and sedation, weight gain, skin rashes, constipation, dry mouth, muscle spasms, rapid heartbeat, blurry vision, and difficult urination.

Withdrawal: Discontinuance must be done at a gradual pace. Abrupt withdrawal can result in a temporary surge of tardive dyskinesia–like symptoms. Whenever possible, these drugs should be used for short periods of time. Ten to 20 percent of patients using antipsychotics for one year or longer have developed tardive dyskinesia.

This is only a brief glimpse at the new medicines of the mind. I hope it has given you a better understanding of the advances being made in biopsychiatry and psychopharmacology. If your doctor feels that medication is necessary for your teen, he or she will explain in much more detail how and why a particular drug works and how to administer it for optimum results. There is more to therapy, however, than medication. Insight, growth, and confidence can come only from a combination of nonpharmaceutical therapies—including individual, family, and group therapy.

Let's go on to them now—and discover together how a chemical imbalance need not be an excuse not to grow or live up to one's potential. A world of health and greater happiness is waiting.

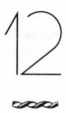

THE THEATER
OF THE MIND

- A study of forty-three adults discovered that over 35 percent of them had psychological problems that were present in childhood.
- Depressed teens stand a greater chance of becoming depressed adults.
- Longitudinal research has found that adult antisocial behavior always begins during the childhood years.
- Only 8.5 percent of the teens in one particular study had psychological problems between the ages of fifteen and twenty-six—because they hadn't experienced any past family problems, such as divorce, loss, death, or separation. But that number jumped to 18.9 percent in teens who had lived through two or more of these childhood traumas.
- A study done at a Detroit clinic found that two years after treatment most of the children suffering from anxiety disorders improved.
- Ninety-one percent of the seventy-two adolescents at a Massachusetts outpatient clinic no longer suffered from anxiety disorders five years after initiating treatment.

- Eighty percent of the people who received psychotherapy at Temple University's outpatient clinic improved—as opposed to only 48 percent of those who decided against treatment.

The evidence is clear: teenagers don't always grow out of their problems. But therapy can successfully help them develop healthfully and normally—and prevent future problems when they become adults.

Today therapy is considered less a luxury and more a necessity among adults coping with the complexities of modern life. The number of adults who have started therapy increases every year.

Unfortunately, therapy for adolescents has not kept up the pace. Although almost 80 percent of the one thousand adults surveyed by the National Association of Private Psychiatric Hospitals strongly agreed that "If you recognized your child to have a mental illness, you'd seek professional help," over 86 percent of these same adults also agreed that "Families find it difficult to admit that their children need professional psychiatric help." As with the sister sciences of biopsychiatry and psychopharmacology, psychotherapy is still shrouded in stigma. This is especially true when it comes to our children, who are the reflections of ourselves and the embodiment of our future.

Child psychiatry's bad reputation can be dated as far back as ancient Greece. Galen, a Greek physician, believed that a person's endowments were set at birth and could be only minimally modified through his or her life. Perhaps it was this erroneous idea that kept infanticide alive up to the nineteenth century. The Middle Ages, too, had no place for adolescence. Youngsters were considered adults by the time they were seven and were literally forced to sink or swim. Happily, this attitude began to change during the seventeenth and eighteenth centuries. A book called *School in Infancy* by Comenius actually offered a parents' sensible guide to child-rearing that included wise instruction, daily exercise, gentle and regulated discipline, and many other principles we still follow today. This more humanistic approach was also advanced by the influential philosophers John Locke and Jean-Jacques Rousseau, who both emphasized the innate goodness and natural development of the child. Chiding, they believed, should be done in private—and praising always a public affair.

The full acceptance of a therapeutic philosophy for children did not take place until 1846, when Edouard Saigine wrote about the "moral treatment" of our troubled young. His doctrine? "Those alone who love them are their true rescuers." We can be our teens' true rescuers—if we are equipped with knowledge, understanding, and an ability to know when help is needed. Drug therapy is only half the story. In the same way that glasses can improve your eyesight, medication can help foster psychological insight and growth in therapy sessions. Together, medication and psychotherapy create the kind of performance that ensures success, the kind that endures with time.

THE MULTIMODAL APPROACH

Adolescent therapies are as varied as their adult counterparts. From individual one-on-one psychotherapy to community support groups that number their members in the hundreds, different types of therapies are available to anyone, in any economic bracket, and in any area of the country. These different therapies are usually combined in a complete treatment "package," called, in psychiatric circles, a multimodal approach. An anxiety-ridden teen might need drug therapy combined with behavioral therapy to help her relax. On the other hand, a teen suffering from an isolated depression triggered by a traumatic event might not need drug therapy at all. His physician might decide that a program of individual and group therapy is sufficient. As variable as the treatment combination might be, there is one constant therapy that is consistently recommended when an adolescent is in pain: family therapy. Because teens live at home with their parents, their problems are both a part of the family's problems and a result—and the insights and skills provided by family therapy are always needed for maximum results.

FINDING THE RIGHT THERAPIST

Only the right medication for an individual teen will work. Similarly, the right relationship between therapist and patient can make all the difference between a treatment that is ineffective and one that works. A therapist who fills every patient's needs is as much a myth as an elusive Superman, but a patient should expect his or her therapist to modify or erase existing symptoms and promote positive growth and development.

THE CHARACTERISTICS OF A GOOD ADOLESCENT PSYCHIATRIST

As detailed in "Cognitive Behavior Therapy with Children and Adolescents" by Paul D. Trautman, M.D., and Mary Jane Rotheram-Borus, Ph.D., in the *American Psychiatric Press Review of Psychiatry*, vol. 7, a good adolescent therapist will aspire to be:

• an active and assertive participant in the therapy process
• responsive, clear, and able to direct the sessions toward an insightful goal
• supportive, while encouraging autonomy within a structured setting
• ready to utilize outside resources, including remedial tutors and support groups
• prepared to emphasize skills training to help a teen better cope with the outside world

To become a therapist takes training. Psychiatrists must complete four years of medical school as well as internships and residency programs. Because they have an M.D., they can prescribe medication. Psychoanalysts, on the other hand, do not need a medical degree. They can be certified social workers, psychiatric nurses, doctors of philosophy, or simply hold a master's degree in psychology in order to receive a license to practice psychotherapy. Because they are not M.D.'s, they cannot prescribe medication. However, they can recommend a drug treatment and work with a psychiatrist who can administer the dosage. Regardless of the degree, if a therapist decides, for example, to specialize in Freudian or behavioral psychology, he or she will need even more years of extensive training. These years of training separate a therapist from a friend. A therapist is skilled in the dynamics of the human mind; he or she understands the techniques involved in treating emotional problems.

A good therapist will:

• Be objective and keep his own values to himself.
• Set up a method of payment to keep the boundaries of the therapeutic relationship formal.
• Continue to be consistent, knowledgeable, and available throughout the therapeutic process.

- Set up an initial interview to help determine whether there is an emotional rapport between patient and therapist.
- Create an atmosphere of trust and support without allowing the patient to become too dependent.
- Help a patient determine when it's time to say good-bye.

Your teen's therapist is at once an ally, a guide, and a teacher. It is as much the therapist's skill as it is the right fit between patient and doctor that will make therapy work, regardless of the therapy of choice. Proof of this comes from a study by Dr. M. B. Parloff et al., which found that a therapist's age, sex, religion, race, experience, or specialization makes no difference to a young patient.

The relationship you and your teen have with a therapist is crucial. But identifying the right therapist also means being familiar with all the varieties of therapy available today. Without further ado, let's go over each one of these different therapies. By the end of this section, you will better understand this theater of the mind that makes hope—and long-term health—a reality for all.

THE MYSTERY UNRAVELED, OR PSYCHOTHERAPY

Images of dark-paneled walls and muted lighting. The silent therapist taking voluminous notes as the patient talks. The patient lying on a couch, ruminating on the past. To many people, this is psychotherapy. Perhaps in Freud's time this was the reality. But today, the world of psychotherapy is different.

The above scenario is really a portrait of traditional Freudian psychoanalysis, which attempts to "make the unconscious conscious." Although adolescent psychiatrists do make use of Freud's developmental theories (see chapter one), his methodology is used less widely. Time-consuming and expensive, psychoanalysis requires patience and extreme introspection—two things adolescents have in short supply. Further, it doesn't always give a person the skills needed to act in healthier ways.

Contemporary therapists are more eclectic. Like the scenes depicted between the troubled, suicidal boy and his therapist in the movie *Ordinary People,* today's therapy sessions are more informal. Patients and therapists sit on comfortable chairs; they face each other and engage in active conversation. Sessions are held only once or twice a week and, unlike during strict psychoanalysis, the present is considered as important as the past.

Freud's legacy does live on in psychotherapy's basic tenets. Emotions are key. They are the elements that, if examined and analyzed, will unlock and ultimately release the pain a teen is feeling. Psychotherapy allows a patient to reexperience the traumatic events that set off his disorder in a safe environment. Through this "abreaction," the troubled teen can discover why the event caused so much pain—and how his feelings and his behavior were affected. He can finally mourn the loss and get on with life.

Exploration of the past is necessary in psychotherapy because adolescents are still developing. The way they reacted to an event when they were six is different than if it had happened in the present. But the troubled teen still reacts in the same way she did when she was six. Here's an example: Jason was five when his parents divorced. He was traumatized at that time and believed it was his fault. At this stage of his development, he felt as if his world had been ripped in two. He began to feel worthless; his view of the world became hopeless and he felt helpless. Now, at sixteen, Jason is once again devastated because his girlfriend has broken up with him. His world has been ripped apart a second time. The feelings he'd been carrying around with him since he was five have been reinforced and reconfirmed—and he continues to believe in his dark view of a pain-filled world. Jason cannot put losing his girlfriend into its proper perspective because of the developmental problems he suffered so many years ago.

Some of the techniques used to find these buried, complex emotions have also evolved since Freud's time. They include the scenarios of:

FREE ASSOCIATION. Rick, a depressed teen, has started talking about the spring—which had come to mind when he saw the sun through the therapy office windows. He wishes it was spring. But he suddenly associates the idea of spring with his brother, who died last May. The therapist gently encourages him to continue talking. "What does it feel like? What are you feeling right now as you talk about this painful time?" She helps him focus in on the traumatic event, helping him gain valuable insight on the experience via his emotional state.

DREAM INTERPRETATION. Rick has been encouraged to keep a notebook of his dreams. He writes them down and brings them to his therapy sessions. Today, he particularly wants to discuss the dream he had last night, a dream in which his schoolbooks came alive, laughing and jeering and taunting him. The therapist guides him through the dream, nodding and interrupting him. She makes a suggestion. Maybe Rick has been taking too much on at school; maybe he should stop trying so hard until he feels better. She provides the reassurance Rick needs to hear in order to slow down.

TRANSFERENCE. Rick has been in therapy for several months, and a trusting relationship has been built. The therapist has taken on the role of his parent—which allows the therapeutic process to enter vulnerable territory. Rick begins to discuss his anger toward his mother, how she sometimes refuses to talk to him, and how he's certain she blames him for his brother's death. Unlike Rick's mother, the therapist listens; she is consistent; she discusses the situation in his home. She is the understanding mother, and she encourages him to talk. She tells him that perhaps his mother too is suffering and is not feeling too nurturing right now. Rick nods his head. He is listening; there is no need to act defensive or feel guilty with his therapist mother. What she is saying makes sense and sinks in.

RESISTANCE. Things have progressed now at a steady clip. But Rick is starting to feel uncomfortable. He and his therapist have begun talking about the anger he feels toward his brother. It's too sensitive a subject; he feels threatened. Rick is afraid to discuss his feelings with his therapist, this person he has grown to trust. What if she abandons him too? Instead, he grows angry and says, "You're just like my mother. You don't really care!" He starts coming to his sessions late. His therapist, however, continues to remain consistent and logical. She doesn't return his anger. And, more important, she doesn't abandon him. Instead, she guides Rick into talking about his feelings, about his fears. He begins to understand. He begins to accept his brother's death. He begins to grow.

Of course, the process of psychotherapy is not as simple as these examples make it seem. It is a complex interaction between patient and therapist, a mixture of problem-solving, insightful growth, education, caring, and support. True psychotherapy is a mourning process in which a teen ultimately accepts and copes with an imperfect world. He learns to deal with the stress that triggered his distress. He no longer uses his disability or genetic predisposition as an excuse to act out. He accepts that his parents are not completely perfect. He discovers that his perceptions of his past have been distorted. He finds that the negative picture he had of himself was false. He learns to take responsibility for his actions and no longer use his disorder to avoid life and all that it has to offer. In short, psychotherapy releases the inner demons that have colored and distorted a teen's view of the world. Like a positive Pandora's box, it introduces a teen to a future filled with hope.

CRIMES OF THE HEARTH, OR FAMILY THERAPY

Family bonds run deep. All of us are tied to our families—sometimes with anger, sometimes with warmth, sometimes with real pain. The love a teenage girl didn't receive as a child. The neglect a teenage boy experienced as a toddler. The sexual abuse a teenage girl had to live with before reaching puberty. We all want a loving, caring family, but we must accept the harsh reality of not having it if we don't. Within the family circle, we can all learn how to be more loving, caring, and more close-knit.

That's where family therapy comes in. We have already seen the role a family plays in a child's development—from biological structure to socialization, from the critical unfolding of self to mastering cognitive tasks. We have also seen the family's pervasive—and persuasive—power and its need to maintain a balance at all costs. It's a cost that can carry a price tag of denial, scapegoating, and a loss of love. Family therapy recognizes that both the troubled teen and the family react with each other to create the initial problem as well as new ones. To alleviate these problems, there are several different methods therapists use in family therapy. These include:

THE STRUCTURAL OPEN-SYSTEMS FRAMEWORK. This therapeutic model holds that family problems are a result of miscommunication. Each family has its system, and each member within this system has a specific role, relationship, and function that influences the other members. As life goes on, the system itself changes, dynamically reflecting the different transitions of family life—from marriage and birth to the children's leaving the nest. By concentrating on the communication problems that can crop up during each transition, these therapists feel the dysfunctional behavior will automatically stop.

Here's an example: Jane was very depressed and stayed in her room all day and night. Her parents were furious. They didn't know this strange adolescent; they didn't know what had happened to their good little girl. They grew frustrated and impatient. Consequently, Jane fell deeper and deeper into her depression. In family therapy, Jane learned to discuss her complex, new feelings with her parents. They responded in turn and explained how they felt. Both began truly to communicate with each other—for the first time. Frustration abated; there were no more angry words. Jane began to feel better.

THE LEARNED BEHAVIORAL APPROACH. Here, the focus is on the rewards and punishments that are consciously or unconsciously given out in a

THE STRESS CALLED MOVING

Moving is one of life's great stresses—for everyone in the family. Unfortunately, parents can unwittingly make relocation more stressful for their teens. The pressure and guilt they themselves are feeling make for denial. Instead of allowing teens to express their fears and loss, parents will negate them with words of encouragement like, "You'll love this new place. It's great. There's a wonderful school and you'll make lots of new friends. Stop acting so mopey. You'd think you were going to jail!" If parents shared their own anxieties and fears about the move with their teens, everyone would feel better, and depression might never have a chance to take hold.

family. It is this punishment/reward system that keeps control in the hands of a specific family member—as well as reinforces negative behavior in a dysfunctional family group. A therapist using this method tries to change the way a family interacts by changing this punishment/reward system.

To illuminate: Margot had an eating disorder. Her parents were constantly telling her to eat—without realizing that, in giving her all that attention at the dinner table, they were actually rewarding her starvation. Instead, the therapist suggested that Margot's parents ignore her when she didn't eat—and reward her with praise when she did.

THE PSYCHODYNAMIC MODEL. This goes beneath the surface to reveal the unconscious dynamics of a particular family, dynamics that have been passed on from generation to generation. If, for example, an anxiety-disordered teen's mother had separation problems when she was young, she can unconsciously pass her fears on to her child. As the expression "Like mother, like daughter" goes, since her first role model used dysfunctional child-rearing practices, she in turn might use the same methods herself.

THE DIFFERENTIATION MODEL. First formulated by Dr. Gary L. Bowen, this view sees the family as a great mass of undifferentiated humanity, from which individuals hatch and become unique. But this can only occur when the families are attuned to the process of separation and individuation. In healthy families, this process occurs naturally. But dysfunctional families must learn through therapy how to hatch their offspring—regardless of a child's age.

Many teens have family problems because they couldn't separate from their parents. Despite being abused or neglected, they still couldn't let go and become separate individuals. A case in point is a girl in the Performance Group who was abused by her natural parents and, at nine, was put in a foster home. Today she not only has to deal with the problems the abuse inflicted, but she also still wants to know why her natural parents abandoned her. She wants them to take her back. Like a child whose parents have divorced, she keeps fantasizing that they will come for her with loving arms. To become healthy she must learn to give up this dream and accept the world and her parents as they are—and accept herself as a separate, unique individual.

IF A TEEN HAS ATTEMPTED SUICIDE, A THERAPIST MUST:

Reason with her . . .
Let her know that the way she is feeling is not permanent, and that with the right help her problems can be worked out.
Stress the facts . . .
and let her know that you are there for her.
Inform . . .
the teen that society looks on suicide as a weakness and remind him of the impact his tragic death would have on his family.
Interfere . . .
with the patient's social life in any way possible to ensure that the teen speaks to her therapist before attempting suicide again.
Include . . .
the patient's entire household in making sure all methods of suicide are guarded against in the home.
Admit to the hospital . . .
any teen who is in imminent danger of taking his own life.

THE PARADOXICAL APPROACH. The best way to explain this methodology is through an anecdote from *Beginning Child Psychiatry* by Drs. Paul L. Adams and Ivan Fras: George Fox, a Quaker in the early days of our country, was in the midst of a discussion with the legendary William Penn. Although Penn considered himself a nonviolent Quaker, he could not give up the sword he kept at his side. This inconsistency confused him. Fox simply said, "I would advise you to go on carrying your sword as long as you can." There was a pause. And Penn promptly gave up his sword.

Paradoxical approach therapists believe that if you put family members into a paradoxical situation, they will change their dysfunctional behavior. You might say they are asked to put their stress to the test. For instance, the therapist might tell the family to go ahead and argue—but at a specific hour of the day or night. The therapist would also tell them when to stop. By arguing "on schedule," a family learns that a seemingly uncontrollable event—a family argument—can be controlled. Family members learn that they don't have to argue, and with the help of a therapist they can learn more constructive ways to express their anger. The impact each family member has on the others is only part of the reason family therapy is necessary. Other reasons include:

- The teenager's problems have created a great deal of tension in the family—and that stress must also be treated.
- The parents might be in need of therapy themselves—for depression or alcoholism or generalized anxiety.
- A family has to know and understand what is going on with their teenager. Their prejudices against therapy, their own problems, their fear of change, and even their good intentions, might inadvertently sabotage a teen who is on the road to recovery.

Family therapy is a powerful tool. Witness the example of a study of twenty-six schizophrenics who were released from a psychiatric hospital. Eighteen of them had families who received family therapy, including instructions on coping, expressing their emotions, and finding new ways to solve problems that might come up at home. After nine months, only one of these eighteen had been readmitted into the hospital—as opposed to eight from the group who didn't have family therapy. Another study of agoraphobic teens found that parents' participation actually helped to eradicate the disorder. As symptoms decreased the family relationship improved. Family therapy is clearly a crucial ingredient of a treatment program's success.

THE ACTION ADVENTURE, OR BEHAVIORAL THERAPY AND SOCIAL SKILL TRAINING

No parent is a stranger to behavioral therapy: Every time you turned a deaf ear to your toddler's temper tantrum, praised the school project your child spent hours putting together, or emphatically said, "No! Don't touch that!"—all these are techniques used in behavioral therapy. Behavioral therapy revolves around the stimulus/response mechanism. By either changing the way we respond to environmental stimuli or changing the stimuli themselves, behaviorists believe we can change the way we act. The parents of an overweight depressed girl can help keep her weight under control by removing fattening (and stimulating) foods from the house. The teacher of a boy suffering from ADHD can respond by ignoring him when he runs around the room. The parents of an unhappy learning disabled boy can have him transferred to a special school environment where he won't feel like a failure. While psychotherapists deal more with the why—the internal, unconscious motives that they believe govern our behavior—behavioral therapists deal with the how, the actions of a teenager in the here and now.

It all began with Pavlov's dogs in the beginning of this century. By ringing a bell at the same time that he brought them food, Pavlov eventually taught his dogs to salivate at only the sound of the bell, thus proving that the response to a stimulus can be learned. Pavlov's basic tenets were refined and developed over the decades, from Watson's theory that, rather than being from the heart, emotions are really conditioned responses to outside stimuli, to Skinner's belief that responses are reinforced by punishments and rewards—a concept still widely used today.

Behavioral therapy has a lot of appeal—especially for adolescents. It is fast and focused. It deals with the present instead of delving into the past. And it has results. Follow-up studies of families who received behavioral-oriented treatment showed vast improvement a full year after the therapy stopped and success that surpassed the more traditional forms of therapy.

Still, behaviorism remains controversial, and there are professionals who object to it. One group feels that the laws of learning that worked in the laboratory are too simplistic to work in the real world. In contrast, another group fears that behaviorism works so well that a few people could end up controlling and manipulating the masses. In reality neither end of the spectrum is correct. When combined with other forms of therapy, behaviorism can replace dysfunctional responses—such as phobias, compulsions, and depressive viewpoints—with positive ones. Here's a brief sampling of how:

SIGNING CONTRACTS. This can mean anything from a letter of intent, in which an anorexic girl promises her therapist she will gain one pound a week, to a written agreement whereby a depressed boy promises to ask a loved one, "Why do you like me?" whenever a dysfunctional, negative thought creeps into his mind.

INSTILLING PUNISHMENTS AND REWARDS soon after the action. One way this works with conduct-disordered teens is via a "point system." On a chart his parents keep a boy receives a point every time he thinks before he acts impulsively, every time he goes to school, every time he stops himself from yelling at his sister. Points are subtracted whenever his behavior gets out of hand. Another device for punishment is a "time out" room, a place where the boy must stay for, say, fifteen minutes every time he acts out. Usually a safety-proofed bathroom or laundry room, this "time out" area immediately stops disruptive behavior and allows parents to take charge of the situation. A reward, on the other hand, could be fifteen minutes' more television or a fifteen-minute extension of curfew.

ROLE MODELING. Teenagers learn by imitating. If a therapist is someone they admire, they will try to act like her. To encourage this, a therapist will always act in a consistent and supportive manner. She might offer positive events from her own life and discuss how she found a positive solution to a problem.

SYSTEMATIC DESENSITIZING. This is a stage-by-stage process in which a fearful situation is turned into a neutral one. Beginning with a mild anxiety-producing stimulus, a therapist using systematic desensitizing will gradually build up to a worst-case scenario. At each stage, a phobic teen realizes she has survived; by the time she is exposed to her most horrible nightmare she has been literally desensitized to the experience. Desensitizing is either done in vitro, in which slides or hypnosis are used to re-create the phobic situations, or in vivo, in which the situation is actually experienced in small doses. Here's an example:

Mike was terrified of fish. His therapist treated his phobia by first showing him a slide of a goldfish in a bowl. He gradually built up to a slide of a great white shark swimming in the ocean. Marie, too, was afraid of fish. But her therapist used actual experience. He had her look at a goldfish bowl for ten minutes. Later, he took her to an aquarium. And, finally, he had her swim in a lake where fish were plentiful. Research has found that in vivo desensitizing is usually more effective. In one study, a group of teens suffering from a swimming phobia was given in vivo desensitizing; a second group was treated with in-vitro methods. The teens who actually went into the water were more successful in neutralizing their fear.

Sometimes painful stimuli are combined with pleasurable ones to get the desired result—an "emotive imagery" technique that, in one study, cured seven out of nine youngsters suffering with phobias. One of the successful seven was a fourteen-year-old boy who was terrified of dogs but adored Alfa-Romeos. Drs. A. A. Lazarus and A. Abramovitz had him imagine himself in his beloved sports car—while interacting with dogs.

RELAXATION. As with their adult counterparts, stressed-out teens must learn to relax. Not only is a relaxed state important for techniques like systematic desensitizing to sink in, but relaxation is an effective therapy in its own right. A teenager who learns the process of self-hypnosis, meditation, or deep breathing can often keep an anxiety attack at bay.

Therapists using relaxation techniques will also teach their teenage patients how to become more attuned to their bodies. Exercise is not only an effective way to release pent-up anxiety, it also helps a teen understand his physiology and gain some control over his stress.

Thanks to the proliferation of Walkmans, cassette tapes have become another valuable tool. Programmed with positive messages and relaxation techniques, they can be used at home—reinforcing what a teen has learned in his sessions. Sometimes descriptive imagery is also incorporated into these tapes. Here, the teen, her eyes closed, her muscles relaxed, visualizes herself on, say, a sailboat skimming gently across the water. She becomes calm, and her breathing slows. Within fifteen minutes, the tape ends and she wakes up refreshed. By learning any of the techniques of relaxation, anxious teens can gain valuable control over their out-of-control anxiety.

COGNITIVE THERAPY. Listen to this dialogue between a therapist and Tony, his eleven-year-old patient:

Therapist: Tony, you said one of your problems is you're stupid.
Tony: Yes, I am.
Therapist *(not attempting to refute this):* When you think, "I am stupid," how do you feel?
Tony: Bad. And sad.
Therapist: Uh-huh. I would feel that way too if I believed I was stupid. *(Labeling the thought)* "I'm stupid" is an automatic thought. It's negative and absolute. Let's talk about it and see if we can figure out if it's true.
Tony: It is true.
Therapist: Well, you may be right. But I don't know you very well yet so I'm just not sure. Let's gather some facts about it.
Tony: What kind of facts?
Therapist: Well, you said, "I'm stupid," or "I think I'm stupid." What made you say that?
Tony: The social worker told me it's not that I am stupid but that I think I am.
Therapist: Well, which is it?
Tony: I'm not sure.
Therapist: Good, then we'll try to figure it out together.*

This therapy session utilizes cognitive therapy, a branch of behaviorism that interjects a crucial element between stimulus and response: thought. Cognitive therapists believe that thoughts govern our moods. If a patient can change the way he thinks, he can change the way he feels and, subsequently, the way he acts—regardless of outside stimuli.

Cognitive therapy has had a great deal of success among teens suffering from depression. Through various techniques, including written homework assignments, record-keeping, charts, and role-playing, the cognitive therapist will rationally and logically help a teen stop thinking in negative ways. To further ensure success, the therapist will always involve the family—whose own faulty reasoning often perpetuates the patient's depressive thoughts. From the same article in which the above cognitive therapy session appeared, here's an example of a cognitive therapy technique in action:

*Excerpted with minor changes from "Cognitive Behavior Therapy with Children and Adolescents" by Paul D. Trautman, M.D., and Mary Jane Rotheram-Borus, Ph.D., in the *American Psychiatric Press Review of Psychiatry,* vol. 7.

Name: Jim R. *Age:* 17 *Date:* 5/1/86

Event: Playing guitar in the basement with Rob and Eddie. Trying to make up a new song. They're just messing around, not serious. Drank some beer.

Feelings/emotions (rate strength 0–100): disappointed (60), discouraged (50), tired (82), depressed (75).

Automatic thoughts: I can't talk to them; I'm dead; I don't feel like doing anything anymore.

Behaviors (what happened next?): Told them I wanted to watch football so I wouldn't have to hang out with them anymore; they left; went to sleep.

Goals (desired outcomes): Make up a new tune; practice with Rob and Eddie; tell them what I want to do; talk to them, just an easy conversation.

Alternative thoughts: When Eddie doesn't talk, it's harder for me to talk; beer makes me feel worse; when things don't work out the way I want them to, I often feel tired; I made up a song last week, it was pretty good.

Alternative behaviors: Tell them I never want to see them again; tell them off; tell them I want to really practice for an hour, then we can hang out someplace; find some new guys to play with; quit guitar.

Costs and benefits (advantages/disadvantages): They're the best friends I've got!; they might not listen; a new bass player would improve the band—Rob's not very good and not motivated.

Plan of action, final outcome: Practice again on Wednesday night; played my new tune, Eddie's a great drummer; only a little depressed (40), not tired at all, Eddie still doesn't talk much.

As this example proves, cognitive therapy's direct and active examination of a teen's distorted view of the world ultimately opens up a more realistic—and positive—world.

SOCIAL SKILLS TRAINING. From taunting classmates to always sitting on the bench during athletic events, from continuous dateless weekends to unfriendly stares in the high school hall, interpersonal relationships cause a great deal of pain to many teens. Behaviorists believe that if, say, a shy girl is taught to venture out of her shell, she will gain needed confidence in herself. She will also find that the support and friendship of others helped change her negative self-image. How is this done?

Through a therapist's coaching, teaching, and reinforcing through a reward system.

Through social skill training, a teenager can learn how to be more:

- Assertive in all her relationships.
- Considerate and polite to other people.
- Attentive to the feelings and behaviors of her peers and parents.
- Confident in social situations.

Whether it's as complex as helping a very troubled teen overcome aggressive behavior that turns others off, or as simple as giving a teen the rudiments of making introductions, saying hello, or trying out the new dance steps, social skill training offers teens a sense of competency in the outside world and gives them the tools they need to cope with life.

Education, too, has its place in skill training. Remedial reading and math, exercises to circumvent learning disabilities, special programs and facilities—all these can make the difference between a learning disabled teenager who gives up and one who copes with the real world, with success.

ALL TOGETHER NOW, OR GROUP THERAPY

Nadine had hit an impasse in her individual therapy. She was having difficulty expressing her insecurity about other people. She believed not only that she was disliked—but that she was disliked because she was a terrible person. When Nadine started group therapy, she discovered there were other kids who felt the same way she did. Further, she found that they were likable, and that their negative views of themselves were in reality completely wrong. If they were wrong about people not liking them, well, perhaps she was wrong, too.

There is safety—and strength—in numbers. Group therapy can reinforce the insights a teenager discovers in individual therapy. It can provide valuable social skills as this same teen begins to interact with others. It can create a secure environment of peer support—especially for the hesitant newcomer to therapy.

In his book *The Theory and Practice of Group Psychotherapy,* Irvin D. Yalom lists the eleven elements of group therapy that make it work:

- *Installation of hope.* A close connection with other teens who are also struggling toward adulthood provides inspiration, strength— and the hope that things can change.
- *Universality.* By listening to the experiences of others in the group, a troubled teen realizes she is not alone—and that others understand her pain.
- *Imparting of information.* Group therapy is almost a classroom in minature, where only relevant subjects are taught. By explaining the therapeutic process, discussing the physiological effects of depression, or pointing out the reasons for hyperactivity, the therapist helps the group find concrete understanding and better control over their problems.
- *Altruism.* By offering the other group members advice, strategies for coping, sympathy, and encouragement, a troubled teen learns firsthand that he has something valuable to give.
- *The corrective recapitulation of the primary family group.* Call this one-family feeling—which many teens will feel for the very first time within the group. The therapist herself is the supervising parent; the other members of the group complete the family circle. Together, they give a teen the chance to heal old wounds, to discover insights about his real family, to create loving and secure family ties.
- *Development of socializing techniques.* Through the exchange of honest feedback between its members, a group helps members develop important and necessary social skills.
- *Imitative behavior.* We have already seen the value of positive role modeling. In a group, a teenager has the chance to take on bits and pieces of both the therapist and the other members, trying these new selves on for size, evaluating them, then either discarding or internalizing them. As Dr. Yalom writes, "Finding out what we are not is progress toward finding out what we are."
- *Interpersonal learning.* Experience can only be a valuable lesson if it can be clearly discussed, analyzed, and understood. Group therapy, comprised of a trained, supervising therapist and teens who have gone through similar struggles, can provide the ideal environment to learn from the sometimes painful experiences of growing up.
- *Group cohesiveness.* Safety and belonging are both crucial ingredients for growth—and both are found in a group therapy setting.
- *Catharsis.* Within the comfort and security of the group, a teenager

is able to let out the months or years of bottled-up rage, sadness, and confusion. By expressing her real feelings, a teenager will feel a sense of tremendous relief. And she will have made the first step on the journey toward rehabilitation and health.

- *Existential factors.* It's always easier to blame someone else for your problems. A victim cannot change things. A victim cannot even try. Taking responsibility for your own actions and your own feelings translates into mental health. As a member of a group, a teen learns to be a "team player," responsible for others and for himself.

Although these eleven elements concern themselves with formal group therapy sessions, they can also be found in the vast array of support groups available today: Tough Love. Alcoholics Anonymous. Groups for families with learning disabled teens, suicide survivors, single parents—the list goes on.

A MATTER OF LIFE AND BREATH

Here's a deep-breathing exercise both you and your teen can use to help you relax. Try it either lying down or sitting.

1. Take several deep breaths, breathing in through your nose and out your mouth. Close your eyes.
2. Imagine yourself on a deserted beach. The waves are soothing. The sun is bright and warm on your body.
3. Take several more deep breaths as you picture this peaceful scene.
4. You are now going to clench and unclench various parts of your body, clenching as you breathe in, releasing as you breathe out. Start with your eyes, squeezing them shut, move to your jaw, your neck, your shoulders. Continue moving down your body and finish with your toes.
5. Take several more long, deep breaths. Tense your entire body at once—then release. Do this one more time.
6. Open your eyes. You should feel much more relaxed!

Excerpted with minor changes from *Aftershock: Surviving the Delayed Effects of Trauma, Crisis and Loss* by Andrew E. Slaby, M.D., Ph.D., M.P.H. (New York: Villard Books, 1989.)

I don't recommend these support groups as a sole method of therapy for teens (see chapter five), but they are invaluable for reinforcing long-term results as well as supplying needed support and understanding for often overwhelmed and stressed-out parents. Ask your therapist, local hospital, or local community service center for listings of groups in your area. You'll also find names and addresses of various support groups and information centers in the national resources list at the end of this book.

These, then, are the therapies that make up the theater of the mind, the vehicles that, when combined, can bring about dramatic results in the most troubled teen. Therapy, however, is more than "two from column A and one from column B." Merely mixing the different types of therapies together is not enough. For a teen to become truly healthy, two dynamics must be dealt with at once.

THE CIRCLE GAME

Call the disorder and the situation that caused it the outer circle of pain. A skillful therapist will use any means available to treat this illness— from medication to social skills training. But there is an inner circle of motivating pain that must be treated as well. The therapist must also penetrate this inner circle, delving deeper and deeper, until the place where the teen's distorted, negative view had given birth is found. Ultimately, it is acceptance of the events that caused this negativity that matters. Accepting who he is. Handling his strengths and coping with his weaknesses. Understanding how he came to suffer from his distortions and negativity. Unleashing the demons that have preyed on his lack of hope, confusion, and pain. With that acceptance, both circles will disappear and a teen will be free to grow, to dream, to simply live a life without pain.

But sometimes a teenager's pain reaches crisis proportions, and hospitalization is needed.

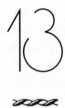

THE HOSPITAL SETTING

The doorways of the rooms that line the deserted corridor are festooned with wreaths and ribbons. At the end of the corridor is another doorway framing a Christmas tree bathed in light. As you walk down the corridor you begin to hear the soft strum of a guitar, the sound of voices singing. Entering the room, you see the source of the music: Thirty young patients, ranging in age from twelve to nineteen, are gathered informally on the floor around the tree. They have just begun singing "The First Noel," accompanied by Elaine Hatala, their recreational therapist, on the guitar. The room they are in is decorated with Christmas drawings, holly, and opened presents; a nearby table holds cookies, punch, and fruit. Sitting on chairs near the patients are staff members, watching the teenagers' performance. As "The First Noel" winds down, a fifteen-year-old girl gets up from the floor. She's wearing jeans and a bright green sweater. Her long blond hair is tied back with a red ribbon. She looks down at the piece of loose-leaf paper in her hand and begins to speak:

Spending Christmas at Fair Oaks Hospital. What a bummer?! But maybe not? After all, the peers and staff of my unit have become my second family and they accepted me just the way I am. It reminds me of a couple years ago, when I spent last Christmas with my grandmother. She lives in California and is very sick. I remember how happy she was to spend Christmas in New Jersey and to be with her family and she also said this would probably be her last Christmas in New Jersey and I didn't take her seriously. But now I realize how lucky I am to be alive and able to spend many more Christmases with my family.

When she is done, the girl looks up and smiles. The staff members applaud and smile back. Elaine Hatala begins the first few chords of "Silent Night, Holy Night." The group begins to sing anew as a few patients casually get up to fetch more cookies. One teen munches on a tangerine. A staff member sips her punch. It's Christmas Eve at Fair Oaks Hospital and the place is filled with spirit. And, if there is some sadness and pain, it is mixed with a lot of hope.

The majority of these teens now consider themselves lucky—although when they first entered the hospital, they were confused, angry, resentful, and scared. As one of my patients told me, "I felt like I didn't need it, you know. Like, I don't need to be here." An outside observer could easily see beyond this denial. Attempted suicide. Violence. Substance abuse. A psychotic episode. When a teen is in danger of harming himself or others, emergency intervention in a controlled environment is necessary. Security and support are available twenty-four hours a day—not only to help circumvent the drug overdose or the self-mutilation, but to provide an objective, consistent atmosphere where the underlying disorders that led to the crisis can be addressed and treated.

A hospital stay can also be recommended when there has been no one crisis, no one disturbing or dangerous incident. A severe depression. A long-term school phobia. Acute anorexia nervosa. Any of these disorders can reach a point of no return, a place where pain and frustration can simply not be tolerated anymore—both in the parents and in their teens alike.

LEGAL TENDER

Hospitalization can be abused. It can mean the loss of liberty and constitutional freedom. In 1979 the United States Supreme Court upheld a Georgia court ruling that said that a neutral fact finder, such as a director of a hospital, is protection enough against unnecessary hospitalization. The Court believed that the parents' action springs from good intentions and that their physician could determine whether or not their teen needs to be hospitalized. Some states, however, do require judicial hearings for adolescents. At Fair Oaks Hospital, every patient under eighteen must appear before a judge at regular intervals during their hospital stay. They always have the right to sign a seventy-two-hour notice of discharge as well as the right to refuse to take their medication. Conduct-disordered teens who have been placed in a hospital by a courtroom judge as an alternative to incarceration do not have these same liberties. Instead, these teens meet with a court-appointed official or parole officer on a regular basis.

THE SILVER LINING

Unfortunately, as positive an experience as a hospital stay can be, it is often seen in a negative light—and as a place beset by failure and hopelessness. In fact, a survey of one thousand adults by the National Association of Private Psychiatric Hospitals felt that "it puts a cloud over this person's head for the rest of his/her life" when a teen is admitted to a psychiatric hospital. Many parents feel tremendous guilt and anxiety when the decision is made to hospitalize their child. And the teen himself can feel his hospital admittance is more a sentence than a cure; he can begin to question his sanity, wondering with terror if he is going crazy.

Although a difficult pill to swallow, hospitalization is frequently the medicine that cures. A hospital stay means a teen can be removed from her stress-filled, triggering environment—whether it be her family or her school. It means that she can deal with her problems without distraction, fulfilling her unresolved developmental tasks and discovering who she is and where she is going—ensuring a sound, well-adjusted future. And it means a complete treatment package that will educate both the teen and the parent—on an intensive, but consistent, supportive, basis.

One of the teens in the Performance Group told me, "I remember when I was like going to bed, I'd feel like, 'This isn't my bed, what am I doing here? Why do I have to be here?' And then I'd start to cry. I'd get all upset about being at a hospital. Then I'd get mad at myself for doing the thing I did in outpatient, that I'd just wasted my time, the whole time." This boy was admitted to Fair Oaks Hospital for a major depressive episode combined with a conduct disorder. None of his previous treatments had proven successful. But eighteen months of hospitalization has done what outpatient therapy has not: It has helped him become a productive and well-adjusted member of society. He is graduating from high school this June and plans to go to college.

Eventually, a troubled teen will settle down into the hospital's routine. She will become healthier, and the better she feels, the less anxiety and guilt her parents will feel. Despite its negative connotations, a hospital provides not only professional and experienced knowledge of adolescence and its disorders, but also an entire range of solutions tailor-made to fit the individual teen. Rather than the end of a long, bitter, and rocky road, hospitalization can be the beginning of a new, exciting journey—for everyone in the family.

TIME IS ON ITS SIDE

"Time heals all wounds." It's an old saying that, though not absolutely true, is an important factor in hospitalization. Time is needed for drug therapy to work. To detoxify a substance-abusing teen. To treat malnutrition resulting from an eating disorder. To build a more positive self-image that prevents future suicide attempts. A hospital stay can mean anywhere from a few weeks to several months or years. The average stay at Fair Oaks Hospital is three months, but the time a teen needs to stay in a hospital varies with each disorder—and with each individual teen.

THE FIRST DAY

"I'll never forget that first day in the hospital, meeting the kids and the staff."

"Going into the doctor's office—that was scary."

"It was like an interview for a job or something. I felt like everyone was looking at me, like they knew where I was going."

"Sure, I was scared. But I was also relieved."

These teens are talking about their admittance into Fair Oaks Hospital. They are not alone in their fear—or their relief. The unknown is terrifying when you're not prepared—and when you are filled with misconceptions and doubts. A well-run institution can go far those first few days in relieving a parent's anxiety and in subduing a patient's fears—especially if you understand exactly how inpatient treatment works. Let's examine what frequently happens when a teenager is admitted to the hospital—and why:

The Initial Interview

"I tried to commit suicide." This was sixteen-year-old Barry's chief complaint—and the reason his parents brought him to Fair Oaks. In my initial private interview with him, I asked him questions regarding his attempt, trying to determine what present-day events triggered his actions—as well as what underlying problems were hidden from view. For Barry, the triggering event was breaking up with his girlfriend of two years because she "didn't like me anymore." I also learned that Barry's parents had had intense marital discord for years—and that Barry often considered himself a pawn in their battles. "They don't love me," he said. "They're only using me." Barry had also begun hanging out with some older kids—and had been using marijuana and smoking cigarettes since he was thirteen. He also had a severe case of acne, which contributed to his low self-esteem.

CUSTODY BATTLE

With the divorce rates climbing, custody battles have become an unfortunate fact of life. Because of the inherent stress and trauma on the children, judges have recently shifted their primary focus to children's needs—and away from the parents themselves. The result is more and more joint custody arrangements. Joint custody can, however, continue a child's trauma and pain if the parents are conflicted or inconsistent. A study of parents who have made joint custody a success found that they had five elements in common:

- Their initial depression and rage did not interfere with their daily work or home routines.
- Their anger was not disruptive or highly intense. Rather than acting out their hostility toward their ex-spouse, they suppressed it.
- Both parents had an essential core of positive self-esteem and self-respect. They trusted themselves.
- They handled their emotions in better ways, tolerating and accepting the ambivalence of simultaneous sadness, anger, and relief.
- They cooperated with each other, focusing on problem-solving instead of emotion. They were open to professional assistance. Agreement was the goal—not revenge.

The initial interview also includes a private session with the teen's parents—not only to determine their point of view, but also to uncover other facts about the teen's development, his relationship with the other family members, and his possible genetic predispositions to a certain illness. When I interviewed Barry's parents, for instance, I learned when Barry first walked and talked, as well as what his early experiences were in school and at home. I also discovered that Barry's father had been severely depressed for years and that his paternal grandfather had been an alcoholic. This psychosocial history helps me draw up a patient's lifeline, which, as I mentioned earlier, gives me a detailed look at the childhood developmental problems that are being addressed again in adolescence, those deep-seated, long-term problems that must be dealt with for success. In Barry's case, his social, self-, and cognitive development had been stymied at the age of five when his father had become depressed—and all his mother's attention was drawn to her spouse. Barry also appeared to have a reading comprehension problem—which also contributed to his negative attitude about school and about himself.

The Evaluation

Is the teen motivated to get well? Are there any physical illnesses that could have contributed to the teen's depressed state? What is the parent's marriage like? Are there sibling problems? Economic problems? Has separation between parent and child taken place? All of these questions go into the complete in-depth evaluation, called a biopsychosocial assessment. The evaluation, done with every teen who enters a hospital, usually takes fourteen days and includes:

A PHYSICAL AND NEUROLOGICAL EXAM. A thyroid problem can look like a depression. So can anemia or malnutrition. In fact, a study of one hundred patients at a mental health center found that 46 percent had a previously undiagnosed medical illness that either accelerated or caused their psychiatric symptoms. And 35 percent of one hundred patients referred to Fair Oaks by their psychiatrists turned out to have an underlying physical reason for their mental pain. To rule out—and treat—a physical illness that is causing a teen's disorder, it is imperative that admitting physicians do a thorough examination.

- *Laboratory testing.* From EEGs to X rays, from metabolic testing to blood workups, laboratory testing helps detect any physical problem—as well as determine if a chemical imbalance is causing a teen's disorder. It gives a physician the facts he or she needs to prescribe appropriate medication.
- *Mental status examinations.* During the initial interviews, a psychiatrist analyzes a teen's social and personal judgment, his memory retention, his ability to understand abstractions. One of the ways physicians at Fair Oaks analyze mental stability is by asking an incoming teen his most important three wishes. Barry answered: "To have clear skin. To find someone to marry who will make me very happy. To make a million dollars so that my mother can live by herself and do what she wants." A telling response.
- *Psychological testing.* Here, the mental status examination is put to the test with in-depth psychological profiles, performance studies, intelligence tests, and more. These tests will also help a physician determine if a learning disability is also a factor in a teen's disorder.

- *A complete medical, psychosocial, and developmental history.* Past and present, an in-depth history of both the teen and her family's dynamics must be taken to help pinpoint the source of a teenager's pain.
- *Consultations* with other specialists or with a teen's school is often necessary to accurately diagnose a patient's problem—and determine a treatment plan. A neurologist would be called in if a teen showed minimal brain damage in his neurological testing. A nutritionist would advise a girl suffering from anorexia nervosa. A school representative would assist the hospital's psychoeducational program in selecting appropriate books and study material for a hospitalized teen.

Like a detective deciphering the clues in a mystery, a physician uses these evaluations to make a differential diagnosis—as exact as possible a diagnosis of the teen's problems. Usually there is more than one disorder that needs to be treated. The predominant ones are labeled AXIS I. AXIS II and AXIS III, influenced by the predominant disorders, follow in descending order. We diagnosed Barry's AXIS I as a major depression, a parent-child problem, and cannabis abuse. AXIS II was a reading comprehension disorder. AXIS III was his acne condition, a contributing factor of his poor self-image.

These Axis diagnoses are like points on a curve; they are dynamic and can change position or disappear during the course of treatment. When Barry's acne cleared up, he no longer had an Axis III diagnosis. Further, when he stopped using marijuana, his cannabis abuse was taken off his Axis I diagnosis—but he continued to need treatment for his major depression.

The Treatment Plan

Most treatment packages are a combination of pharmacotherapy, behavioral therapy, and skill training, and regularly scheduled individual, group, and family therapy. From support group programs to individual one-on-one treatment, a hospital has available many of the same therapies as an outpatient clinic, but all under one roof. There are, however, two therapies I haven't yet discussed because they are primarily used only in a hospital setting: recreational and creative therapy. Both focus more on nonverbal interaction. Creative therapy, for example, uses artwork to teach troubled teens how to express themselves. Drawing and painting encourage teens to open up—which they might not do in more talkative individual or group therapy. They help develop spontaneity and provide a positive outlet for creativity. At Fair Oaks Hospital, we often ask our patients to do a timeline, dividing a piece of paper into threes and doing three different drawings around one theme—with a beginning, a middle, and an end. Some teens used their hospital stay, depicting themselves in a blackened, terrifying place in the first drawing, sketching themselves in a calm, abstract hospital setting for the middle drawing, and, for the end drawing, imagining themselves back out in the world. Some drew flowers or rainbows, while others drew question marks.

Recreational therapies help the troubled teen relax, become more aware of his body, discover new activities for leisure time, and improve social interaction with his peers. Recreational therapy can include everything from volleyball games to field trips to an amusement park. A particular example of a successful recreational therapy is the Performance Group (which you've read so much about throughout this book).

Remedial school sessions are also required to help the troubled adolescent keep up her work during her hospitalization. Instructors trained in dealing with behavioral problems and learning disabilities teach small groups during a regular school day—providing individual attention to deal with a teen's classroom needs. The focus is on the required math, English, social studies, and science, but these subjects are balanced in many hospitals with a number of elective courses, including typing, creative writing, and even driver ed.

The Hospital Routine

At Fair Oaks—and at many other hospitals across the nation—day-to-day operations are based on the Mileau Treatment Program (MTP), a treatment plan of behavior modification that uses a status system and a token economy. Studies have found that this type of treatment plan has a great deal of success. One follow-up study found that teens with conduct disorders who were admitted into a hospital using a behavior modification program had fewer behavior problems, less aggression, and less police involvement and achieved a higher level of independence after two years than those who were not admitted into the program.

Essentially, MTP rewards and reinforces good behavior and punishes the bad. The more points (tokens) a patient receives, the more privileges he can have—eventually working himself up from a Status I to a sought-after and highly independent Status IV. Points are earned, say, for cleaning one's room, for signing a contract to stay off drugs, for being nondisruptive in the hospital school, for actively participating in the different therapies—all of which reinforce positive behavior. Patients can then use their points to listen to the stereo, stay up late Friday nights, see an in-hospital movie, and more. On the other hand, the more disruptively a teen acts, the fewer points she earns—and the fewer privileges she receives.

Another punishment that speaks much louder than words is the Quiet Room—an empty, nonstimulating hospital room used to subdue a teen who has become extremely agitated, abusive, and violent. What makes the Quiet Room so effective is not simply that it is a painless, nonthreatening way to quiet an overstimulated patient down; it's a proven fact that, by reducing the stimulation that can sometimes set off a teen, it helps him gain valuable self-control. A study examining the use of a Quiet Room as a therapeutic tool at the Children's Psychiatric Inpatient Unit at The Johns Hopkins Hospital found it highly successful. Not only was it used less and less as a hospital stay proceeded, but many of the patients asked permission to go into the Quiet Room on their own—taking responsibility for themselves to calm down and regain their self-control.

Psychiatrists, clinical psychologists, clinical social workers, psychiatric nurses, occupational, creative, and recreational therapists, and special education teachers are all a part of a hospital's treatment team, and they all work together to make MTP successful, carrying out its firm and consistent rules and, at the same time, offering twenty-four-hour support, attention, crisis intervention—and valuable feedback. Without feedback, a teen has no idea how well she's doing; she doesn't know how she appears to others.

At Fair Oaks Hospital, we have regularly scheduled meetings in which the entire staff and their adolescent patients gather together, exchanging insights and observations about each other's behavior over the last few days. Twice a week there is a meeting—and twice a week there's a chance for a troubled teen to get feedback and gain insight into his actions. There are also bimonthly meetings of parent education groups and support groups for substance abuse.

Eventually, a teen settles into the hospital routine: breakfast in the morning, school during weekday mornings and afternoons, various therapies after school, business and community meetings during lunch or in the evening, once-a-week Performance Group rehearsals, and, in the evenings, a chance to use the points earned during the day—by watching some television, seeing a movie, or playing pool.

Discharge

Saying good-bye is always difficult, especially for a teen who has grown to love her hospital family, who has made a secure, confident world within the hospital walls. But true health means individuation, separation—and using the tools she learned inside the hospital in the outside world. Discharge is usually done in a ceremonial fashion, with everyone giving their individual good-byes during a special lunch. One member of the Performance Group might tell the departing patient that she has a beautiful voice. Another might say she was a real asset to the group. Still another patient might say she'll be missed. Amid tears and hugs, the departing teen will echo their sentiments of support and love.

Because of the emotionally charged nature of discharge, it must have plenty of advance preparation. There are also practical considerations. Treatment programs must be carefully understood if they are to be followed at home. Medications must continue to be taken. Teens must continue to go to their therapist once or twice a week. Parents and other family members must continue their family therapy.

Further, the teenager herself might regress before the discharge. She might begin to act out again in disruptive, negative ways; she might become tearful, sad, and anxious. These negative emotions and behaviors will usually pass. But a complete evaluation must be done before the teen leaves the hospital to make certain the time is indeed right to say good-bye.

Follow-up

All new healthy habits must be reinforced. Similarly, positive behavior newly learned in the hospital cannot stand alone. Patients and their families are never left stranded once a hospital stay is completed. Not only is there continuous contact through the different outpatient therapies, but, if permission is granted, patients and their parents usually receive phone calls periodically from the hospital staff to see how everyone is doing. Confidential questions regarding family, school and work, friendships, and outpatient therapy help the hospital see how successful their treatment programs are and where improvements might be needed. They also help reassure the patient if he or she is currently experiencing some pain.

Life is not always easy or fair. But hospitalization gives teens who once felt hopeless and helpless a rebirth—and a chance to live life well. As one of our staff members said during a Performance Group good-bye, "I hope that when you go home, things work out for you and that you'll remember what we did here." *That's* what hospitalization is all about. And as a physician I am glad that it can be so successful. But the real goal of every mental-health professional involved in adolescent treatment is prevention—*before* the disorder takes root. Read on to discover how you as parents, your local schools, and your community can together help wipe out adolescent pain.

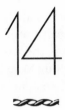

PREVENTION
The Happy Ending

Sometimes problems crop up in the most loving of homes. Even the best of intentions aren't always enough. Despite our love, despite our intelligence and care, our children can have pain. Loving support is one thing, but practical knowledge is another. Together, both can help a parent circumvent the most serious disorder. Together, both can help prevent a problem before it rears its teenage head. Prevention begins at home—starting with the people who have the most impact on a teenager's life: parents.

HOW WELL DO YOU HANDLE YOUR TEENAGER'S "GROWING PAINS"?

Perhaps you believe you've done everything you can. Perhaps you can't think of any other avenues to pursue. Or perhaps you've reached the end of your rope. Whatever you're feeling, the reality that your child has become an adolescent is here to stay. Should you yell at your son to clean his room? Should you listen to your daughter when she tells you to leave her alone? Does your son really like school as much as he claims he does? Is your daughter's staying home on Saturday night a healthy sign of individuality—or a symptom of depression?

In their excellent book *A Parent's Guide to Common and Uncommon School Problems,* psychiatrists Irl Extein and David Gross identify the "Ten Commandments" of good parenting:

1. Improve your communication skills
2. Control your anger
3. Be a problem-solver, not a fault-finder
4. Negotiate agreements
5. Create a consistent, structured environment
6. Present a united front
7. Encourage, don't overwhelm
8. End homework hassles
9. Collaborate with the school
10. Assert your influence

1. Improve Your Communication Skills

Time and time again I have heard teenagers complain that their parents don't listen. It's always the same thing: "My parents don't understand me." "We can't communicate." "They don't talk to me."

Communication is more than a gentle prod. Communication really begins with listening. Dr. Thomas Gordon, in his very influential book *Parental Effectiveness Training (P.E.T.) in Action,* identified four skills of good listening:

- *Passive listening (or silence).* Give your child a chance to speak.
- *Acknowledgment responses.* Even when you're listening passively, it's a good idea to make sincere comments, such as "I see" or "Oh?" that emphasize that you are paying attention. I realize that this seems like simple common sense, but you would be surprised by how many parents will listen silently with a poker face.
- *Door openers.* These are simple and nonjudgmental statements, such as "I was wondering how you felt about going to college." These simple invitations may feel awkward, but they really do serve as an excellent means of "getting the ball rolling."
- *Active listening.* Try restating what your child has just told you, without trying to interject advice or pass judgment. You can, however, try to accent the positive. For example: Your teen: "School stinks. I just can't seem to get the hang of it." You: "Yeah,

the classes you're taking are difficult. But, you know, your grades have improved this year."

Teens want their parents to talk to them; they want to believe they have someone who will listen, who will understand, who will make them feel better.

2. Control Your Anger

Many parents fail to acknowledge the extent of their anger. It is very natural for parents of a troubled teen to be angry at the teen and to be angry at themselves for having "failed" their teenager. Rather than denying this anger, parents should try to deal with their anger in a more constructive fashion. How?

- *Back off.* When you feel yourself getting angry, stop. Don't try to "talk out" your anger with your child. Instead, wait until you've calmed down and then begin the discussion.
- *Think.* Why are you angry at your teenager? Is it something he did, or are you really mad at yourself for something that you failed to do?
- *Understand your emotions.* Anger is often the result of several powerful emotional responses: *fear* that your teen may get hurt, *disappointment* that he or she is not successful, *frustration* over your teen's and your inability to make a quick change, and *embarrassment* over failing as a parent. These emotions, while understandable, often prevent parents from finding constructive solutions.

3. Be a Problem-Solver

If your teen's in trouble, help her; don't wait for her to find her own way out. Now, this doesn't mean thay you should simply impose your solution to the problem. Helping doesn't mean dictating and it certainly doesn't mean criticizing her for failing.

4. Negotiate Agreements

Negotiation is a two-way street: You have to give up something to get something. This doesn't mean that you will have to bribe your teenagers to get them to go to school. It does, however, mean that certain privileges such as a relatively generous allowance or a somewhat flexible curfew will have to be earned. A simple family contract, strictly enforced, will help both the teenager and the parent to reach an agreement. For example, Justin agrees to clean his room once a week in exchange for an extra half hour to stay out on weekends.

5. Create a Consistent, Structured Environment

To those of us who remember the sixties, this may be the most difficult suggestion. After all, we grew up during a time when "doing your own thing" nearly became a trademark for an entire generation. In reality, the permissive attitude of a parent is really just an excuse for bad parenting. Teens need consistency, discipline, guidance, and boundaries. Of course, they will frequently complain about these restrictions, but in reality most teens are glad to know that someone really does care about them. So strong is their need for discipline that some teens, in the absence of adult guidance, will seek out their own sources of discipline through sports, martial arts, or religion.

I encourage parents to establish a time each week for family activities. Saturday afternoon, for example, can be set aside as a "family time" when every member of the family must participate in the activity (whether it be shopping, going to a football game, or watching a movie).

Divorced parents may find a structured schedule difficult to follow, especially around the holidays. For example, consider a typical scenario for a divorced family at Thanksgiving. Both parents want to spend this important holiday with their teenage son, so they decide to be fair and have Johnny spend Thanksgiving afternoon with his mother and Thanksgiving night with his father. Of course, both parents want to have a sumptuous sit-down dinner. Johnny eats well in the afternoon but then has to leave for a rushed trip to his father's house for yet another dinner. Of course, Johnny doesn't feel like eating again and barely picks at his food. Johnny's father and new stepmother misinterpret this lack of appetite as a slap at them. A far better arrangement would have called for Johnny to spend all of Thanksgiving Day with his mother, but the remainder of the weekend with his father.

Often divorced parents will divvy up the holidays on an alternating-year basis ("Last year you had Christmas and Easter while I had New Year's and Thanksgiving, so this year we'll swap"). While this arrangement is equitable for the parents, it can confuse the child and ultimately deprive her of a sense of tradition. I usually recommend that divorced parents *not* alternate holidays from year to year (for example, Christmas should always be spent with Mom and New Year's always spent with Dad). This fixed schedule creates consistency and fosters memories of holiday traditions. These memories can help offset some of the chaotic effects that divorce may bring.

6. Present a United Front

This can be difficult, especially if your teen has become a master at manipulating one parent against the other. However, parents who agree to discuss important matters in private before ruling on their teen's request will severely limit the manipulative talents of their teenager. Divorced parents face an even more difficult challenge: They must agree to not let their problems obstruct their parental responsibilities.

7. Encourage, Don't Overwhelm

Teenagers should be challenged to do better at school, at home, and at sports or hobbies. However, this encouragement should never turn into frustration, or an unrealistic desire for perfection. This is commonsense advice, but, after all, isn't common sense the essence of good parenting?

8. End Homework Hassles

In most families, especially troubled ones, homework is usually a prime battleground. Parents usually want a more dedicated (and successful) approach, while the child resents the intrusion into his free time. Sometimes a parent may be tempted to downplay the importance of homework. Considering the problems of drugs, vandalism, crime, and promiscuous sex, these parents may be relieved if all their child does is stay home and do nothing! In reality, the importance of homework, and the discipline it fosters, should not be underestimated. Remember, homework

- creates a sense of accomplishment
- improves self-esteem
- lets your child know that you think his life and activities are important
- helps your child to feel responsible for his actions

In addition, good homework skills can be taught at any age, and bad homework habits can be broken. To help identify bad homework habits,

Dr. Frederick M. Levine and Dr. Kathleen M. Anesko devised the following homework checklist:

HOMEWORK PROBLEM CATEGORY CHECKLIST*
  1. Doesn't know what homework to do

* Isn't sure exactly what assignment is
* Forgets books or other materials at school
* Completes assignments, but leaves them at home or forgets to hand them in

  2. Doesn't know when to do homework

* Has to be reminded to start homework
* Procrastinates, puts off starting work
* Doesn't work well if alone in room
* Doesn't work well without help (from parents, older brother or sister)

  3. Doesn't know where to do homework

* Doesn't work well if alone in room
* Doesn't work well without help (from parents, older brother or sister)
* Daydreams or plays with things during homework session
* Is easily distracted
* Takes too long to complete homework

  4. Doesn't know how to do homework

* Isn't sure exactly what assignment is
* Whines or complains about work
* Has to be reminded to start homework
* Procrastinates, puts off starting work
* Doesn't work well if alone in room
* Doesn't work well without help (from parents, older brother or sister)

*From the book *Winning the Homework War* by Dr. Frederick M. Levine and Dr. Kathleen M. Anesko © 1987. Used by permission of the publisher, Prentice Hall Press/A division of Simon & Schuster, New York.

- Is easily frustrated by assignments
- Is dissatisfied, even if the work is done well

5. Doesn't know why homework should be done

Defiant:

- Denies having assignments
- Refuses to do assignments
- Is easily frustrated by assignments
- Responds poorly when told to correct work
- Deliberately fails to hand in completed assignments

Unmotivated:

- Fails to bring assignments and materials home
- Whines or complains about work
- Procrastinates, puts off starting work
- Produces messy or sloppy work
- Hurries through work, makes careless mistakes
- Forgets to bring assignment to class

Having identified the problem areas, talk to your teenager and his teacher(s) about possible solutions.

9. Collaborate with the School

Eight hours a day, five days a week—school is such an important part of your child's life that I have devoted an entire section to the subject (see below).

10. Assert Your Influence

While earlier suggestions emphasized the need to improve communication and negotiate agreements, parents should never neglect the importance of their influence and guidance. Parents should always remember to:

- Never be afraid to say "No."
- Make reasonable rules.

- Not threaten your child with punishment that you never intend to carry out.
- Not punish your child unfairly.

Teenagers need your guidance and support at the very moment that they are struggling to break away from you. This dichotomy makes them very vulnerable and susceptible to a wide range of influences. Parents who respond to this vulnerability by withdrawing their guidance are not helping their child. They are only making it easier for their child to succumb to the influences of others.

PREVENTION IN THE CLASSROOM

High school is where we passed that midterm with flying colors—or failed along with others in the class. Where we danced the night away at the junior prom, or stayed at home listening to moody records. Where we cried because we were snubbed by the cool kids in the hall—or joined them on their strut to class. Where we learned a lot more than the ABCs.

School used to be a place where lessons were learned—period. Over the past few decades, we have become more sophisticated—and have acknowledged that much of a child's development occurs within the classroom. A school must provide education by law—but it is just as important for it to offer social and emotional support for a growing teen.

Here's proof: A 1974 study found that, in general, teachers ignore students with behavior problems. They pass them over even if they want to participate in a classroom discussion. Sensitive to the fact that they are being ignored, these students act out even more to get attention. Unfortunately, teachers usually reserve their praise for academic excellence. But if a disabled or conduct-disordered teen follows the rules or acts in an appropriate way—she too should be rewarded. And, as an added bonus, the positive behavior would be enforced.

In his excellent book *Teacher and Child,* Dr. Haim G. Ginott quotes one teacher as saying, "I already know what a child needs. I know it by heart. He needs to be accepted, respected, liked, and trusted; encouraged, supported, activated, and amused; able to explore, experiment, and achieve. Damn it! He needs too much. All I lack is Solomon's wisdom, Freud's insight, Einstein's knowledge, and Florence Nightingale's dedication."

Communities can stop the suicide cluster phenomenon in its tracks. The Centers for Disease Control in Atlanta suggest that your community:

- Formulate a community action plan now, before a suicide cluster begins and panic sets in.
- Avoid sensationalism.
- Identify those teens with high-risk factors and offer them counseling services.
- Alter those places or situations that might cause clustering, such as blocking off a park where suicide attempts are taking place.

Bulleted items reprinted from *High Times/Low Times: The Many Faces of Adolescent Depression* by John E. Meeks, M.D. (Summit, NJ: The PIA Press, 1988).

It's true. To be everything a growing child needs is beyond the scope of a classroom teacher. But schools can work with a teen's parents. They can offer insight into areas not brought up at home. They can provide:

OBSERVATION. Teachers are usually the first ones to catch a learning disability—and early detection means less time for feelings of failure to be instilled. They can also see if aggression is being misplaced—or if a child seems to be depressed and troubled.

TESTING. Education might begin at home, but testing is always done at school. Intelligence tests, achievement tests, school readiness tests, psychological profiles—all of these provide facts to supplement a parent's insights.

SOCIAL SKILLS TRAINING. Melinda, an aspiring doctor, had volunteered to clean out all the cages in the biology lab on Saturday. But by Friday night she was swamped with homework. She learned that she had to go to a family gathering on Sunday. She couldn't possibly clean the cages, do her homework, and go to the affair. Melinda, anxiety-ridden and tearful, went to school on Saturday morning. When she saw her teacher, she explained the situation. The teacher smiled and praised

Melinda's discipline. "With all that going on, you came in anyway. You should feel very proud of yourself. Don't worry about the cages. We'll take care of it another time." Melinda learned a valuable lesson about responsibility and interaction with others. She left school feeling great.

A teacher must teach academic subjects. But she or he can also instill valuable social skills—from respecting others to learning good manners. Teachers can have a tremendous impact.

REMEDIAL EDUCATION. Federal Public Law 94–142 describes special education as "Specially designed instruction, at no cost to parents or guardians, to meet the unique needs of a handicapped child, including classroom instruction, instruction in physical education, home instruction, and instruction in hospitals and institutions." Whether it's a reading comprehension disorder, a conduct disorder, a math block, or simply a lisp, your teen is entitled by law to have remedial education at school.

SUPPORT. Listen to this dialogue from Dr. Ginott's *Teacher and Child:*

Nina: My sister's going to have a baby.
Teacher: You're going to be an aunt.
Nina: Yes, but my sister's not married.
Teacher: Oh.
Nina: Everybody at home was all upset and mad, but I'm happy.
Teacher: You're looking forward to being an aunt.
Nina: Yes, but I wish everyone was happy.
Teacher: You wish they shared your joy.
Nina: Yeah.

Dr. Ginott goes on to write that "Nina paused for a moment, ran over to her teacher, and hugged her." Support can come from many different places.

A PARENT'S BILL OF RIGHTS

The school cannot be expected to solve all your child's problems or carry out your parental responsibilities. Still, you do have a right to ask for the school's cooperation in helping you cope with these problems. (Remember: You shouldn't complain if you haven't asked for the school's help, or if all you do is criticize and blame the teacher!)

- The school should keep you informed about your child's development. If trouble is brewing, you should be told right away, not at the end of the term.
- Homework loads should be regular, not erratic, so you can help your child schedule his time effectively.
- The teacher should be willing to reassess your child's behavior and achievements; he or she may unconsciously assume the child is continuing previous poor behavior patterns even when the child has improved.
- Your child should not feel that he is being singled out, ridiculed, or otherwise discouraged by either the teacher or other students.

Reprinted from *A Parent's Guide to Common and Uncommon School Problems* by David A. Gross, M.D. and Irl L. Extein, M.D. (Summit, NJ: The PIA Press, 1989).

COMMUNICATION BETWEEN PARENT AND TEACHER. In the same way communication is crucial between parent and child, it is vital between parent and teacher. To make a parent-teacher conference effective, parents should approach teachers as allies and not as antagonists. Dorothy Rich, in her fine book *MegaSkills*, suggests that parents:

1. Enter the conference with an open mind and be willing to listen to the what the teacher has to say.
2. Begin the conference with a positive statement about the teacher or school.
3. Inform the teacher of any special circumstances, such as a death in the family or marital problems, that may be affecting the entire family.
4. Discuss in general terms your child's strengths and weaknesses.
5. Then, focus on areas that you think the child needs to improve in.

6. Ask about grades, how they were determined, and where your child stands in relation to the other students.
7. Discuss what you can do to help your child at home.
8. Do not leave any question unanswered (and make certain that you understand the answer).
9. Follow up after the conference and make certain progress has been made.
10. Remember that the teacher's opinion—while important—is only one part of the picture.

The home environment. The classroom setting. Together, they can go far in circumventing teenage pain. But there is still one more area where prevention can do its good work: the community at large.

THE BIGGER PICTURE

"Idle hands are the devil's plaything." This saying might have sent chills up the spines of our Puritan forefathers, but, in slightly different tones, it does have relevance even today. The fact is that the busier a teenager is, the less apt he is to get into trouble.

Football practice. Soccer on Saturday. Piano lessons once a week. Dance class. The Great Books Club. Swim meets and mixers. Supervised field trips. A community center that provides positive recreational activities, keeping teenagers productive and entertained. With school, homework, and these after-school activities, there's no time for trouble. And more important, no need. Communities are also invaluable resources for support. From Alcoholics Anonymous to Tough Love, they can provide the facilities for the support groups that help both parents and teenagers alike.

Preventive measures alone are not always a guarantee that your teen will go through her adolescence without pain. But combined with insight, treatment, and understanding, they can stop a disorder in its tracks. They can keep teenage demons at bay. They can make these years an enjoyable journey—for every member of the family.

As one of the anonymous adults in that community center audience wrote: "I was not left with negative feelings, but rather of hope—hope that I as a parent will keep the lines of communication open and present myself as a positive role model."

That hope is more than half the battle.

EPILOGUE
"There Can Be Changes"

Over 75 percent of the one thousand adults surveyed in that National Association of Private Psychiatric Hospitals survey that I've quoted throughout this book agreed that "you can't generally recognize when a child should see a psychiatrist." This lament was echoed by an anonymous teen in a Performance Group audience who wrote: "What do you do if you have problems which no one realizes?" It is my hope that by the time you read this epilogue you will have developed a better appreciation of your teenager. You will have discovered what it means to be a normal teenager in today's world—and the different ways teenage turmoil can take root. And, most important, it is my hope that you will now recognize the symptoms when your teen is in pain and will know that you can do something about it.

The reasons why teenagers suffer are as varied as the individuals themselves. There is no one factor, no one area to blame. The renowned adolescent psychiatrist Dr. Michael Rutter outlined four different areas that work interdependently, reacting with one another to create a teen's behavior.

The first is individual predisposition, which involves heredity, family dynamics, temperament, and physical illness.

The second is the different social environments, including school, peer group dynamics, and community culture.

The third is the teen's current circumstances, the traumatic and stressful events she or he might be going through.

The fourth is the opportunities that may or may not be open to a teen. A teenage girl might have a history of substance abuse in her family. She might be hanging around with a tough group of kids. She might be suffering from her parents' divorce. But she still won't become a drug abuser if she can't afford the drug—and if it isn't readily available.

The luck of the draw? Perhaps. The dynamics are complex. The disorders that can take root are many, with symptoms that are, at the same time, both universal and unique to the individual teen.

Worthlessness. Making friends. Intense feelings. Family connections. Anger at the world and oneself. These themes come up again and again at Fair Oaks. But as my patients can attest, there are treatments and cures—and prevention for the future.

To grow without fear, without pain, to understand and accept our problems and learn more realistic and better ways to cope, is the goal not only for my treatment program, but for every teen and every adult. The bottom line is always growth. And as William Safire once said, "Below the bottom line is freedom."

May you and your teens always have that freedom.
To grow.
To live productive lives.
To love.
And be loved back.

NATIONAL RESOURCES

American Psychiatric Association
1400 K Street, NW
Washington, DC 20005
(202) 682-6000

National Association of Social Workers
7981 Eastern Ave.
Silver Spring, MD 20910
(880) 638-8799

ATTENTION-DEFICIT DISORDER

Attention-Deficit Information Network (AD-IN)
P.O. Box 790
Plymouth, MA 02360
(508) 747-5180

EATING DISORDERS

The American Anorexia/Bulimia Association
418 East 76th Street
New York, NY 10021
(212) 734-1114

ANAD—National Association of Anorexia Nervosa and Associated
Disorders
P.O. Box 7
Highland Park, IL 60035
(708) 831-3438

ANRED—Anorexia Nervosa and Related Disorders, Inc.
P.O. Box 5102
Eugene, OR 97405
(503) 344-1144

B.A.S.H. (Bulimia Anorexia Self-Help)
66125 Clayton Avenue
Suite 215
St. Louis, MO 63139
(314) 991-BASH

The National Anorexia Aid Society
1925 East Dublin-Granville Road
Columbus, OH 43229
(613) 436-1112

Overeaters Anonymous
World Service Office
P.O. Box 92870
Los Angeles, CA 90009
(213) 542-8363

LEARNING DISABILITIES

Learning Disability Association of America
4156 Library Road
Pittsburgh, PA 15234
(412) 341-1515

Orton Dyslexia Society
724 York Road
Baltimore, MD 21204

MANIC DEPRESSION AND DEPRESSION

Depressives Anonymous
329 East 62nd Street
New York, NY 10021
(212) 924-4979

The Manic and Depressive Support Group, Inc.
15 Charles Street
New York, NY 10014
(212) 533-6374

National Depressive and Manic Depressive Association
53 West Jackson Blvd.
Suite 505
Chicago, IL 60604
(312) 939-2442

SUBSTANCE ABUSE

Al-Anon Family Groups
P.O. Box 862
Midtown Station
New York, NY 10018-0862
(212) 302-7240

Alcoholics Anonymous
General Service Office
Box 459
Grand Central Station
New York, NY 10163
(212) 686-1100

Cocaine Anonymous
P.O. Box 1367
Culver City, CA 90232
(213) 559-5833

Drugs Anonymous
P.O. Box 473
Ansonia Station
New York, NY 10023
(212) 874-0700

Marijuana Smokers Anonymous
1135 South Cypress B
Orange, CA 92666
(714) 997-2926

Nar-Anon Family Group Headquarters
P.O. Box 2562
Palo Verdes, CA 90274-0119
(213) 547-5800

Narcotics Anonymous
World Service Office
P.O. Box 9999
Van Nuys, CA 91499
(818) 780-3951

Pill Addicts Anonymous
General Service Board
P.O. Box 278
Reading, PA 19603
(215) 372-1128

800-Cocaine
P.O. Box 100
Summit, NJ 07901
(800) 262-2463

SUICIDE

The American Association of Suicidology
2459 South Ash
Denver, CO 80222

Survivors of Suicide (S.O.S.)
3251 N. 78th Street
Milwaukee, WI 53222
(414) 442-4638

SOURCES

Adams, Paul L., M.D., and Fras, Ivan, M.D., *Beginning Child Psychiatry.* New York: Brunner/Mazel, 1988.

Agras, W. Stewart, and Kirkley, Betty G., "Bulimia: Theories of Etiology," *Handbook of Eating Disorders: Physiology, Psychology, and Treatment of Obesity, Anorexia, and Bulimia,* ed. by Kelly D. Brownell and John P. Foreyt. New York: Basic Books, Inc., 1986.

Alessi, Norman E., Robbins, Douglas R., and Dilsaver, Steven C., "Panic and Depressive Disorders Among Psychiatrically Hospitalized Adolescents," *Psychiatry Research,* no. 20, 1987.

American Psychiatric Association, *Facts About: Teen Suicide.* (pamphlet) Washington, D.C.: American Psychiatric Association, 1988.

Bailey, George W., M.D., and Egan, James H., M.D., "Conduct Disorders," *American Psychiatric Press Review of Psychiatry,* vol. 8, Allan Tasman, M.D., Robert E. Hales, M.D., and Allen J. Frances, M.D., eds. Washington, D.C.: American Psychiatric Press, Inc., 1989.

Barlow, David H., and Seidner, Andrea L., "Treatment of Adolescent Agoraphobics: Effects on Parent-Adolescent Relations," *Journal of Behavior Research and Therapy,* vol. 21, no. 5, 1983.

Barrett, Mark E., Simpson, D. Dwayne, and Lehman, Wayne E. K., "Behavioral Changes of Adolescents in Drug Abuse Intervention Programs," *Journal of Clinical Psychology,* vol. 44, no. 3, May 1988.

Barrymore, Drew, "The Secret Drew Barrymore," *People,* January 16, 1989.

Berg, Ian, Butler, Alan, Faibairn, Irene, and McGuire, Ralph, "The Parents of School Phobic Adolescents—A Preliminary Investigation of Family Life Variables," *Psychological Medicine,* no. 11, 1981.

Berkovitz, Irving H., "Aggression, Adolescence, and Schools," *Adolescent Psychiatry,* vol. 14, 1987.

Berlant, Jeffrey L. M.D., Ph.D., Extein, Irl, M.D., and Kirstein, Larry S., M.D., *Guide to the New Medicines of the Mind.* Summit, NJ: The PIA Press, 1988.

Blau, Gary M., M.S., Gillespie, Janet F., Ph.D., and Evans, Elizabeth G., Ph.D., "Predisposition to Drug Use in Rural Adolescents: Preliminary

Relationships and Methodological Considerations," *Journal of Drug Education,* vol. 18, no. 1, 1988.

Bonaguro, John A., Ph.D., Rhonehouse, Michael, B.A., and Bonaguro, Ellen W., Ph.D., "Effectiveness of Four School Health Education Projects Upon Substance Abuse, Self-Esteem, and Adolescent Stress," *Health Education Quarterly,* vol. 15, no. 1, Spring 1988.

Boskind-White, Marlene, and White, William C., Jr., "Bulimarexia: A Historical-Sociocultural Perspective," *Handbook of Eating Disorders: Physiology, Psychology, and Treatment of Obesity, Anorexia, and Bulimia,* Kelly D. Brownell and John P. Foreyt, eds. New York: Basic Books, Inc., 1986.

Brent, David A., M.D., Perper, Joshua A., M.D., L.L.B., M.Sc., Goldstein, Charles E., A.C.S.W., Kolko, David J., Ph.D., Allan, Marjorie J., Allman, Christopher J., and Zelenak, Janice P., Ph.D., "Risk Factors for Adolescent Suicide: A Comparison of Adolescent Suicide Victims with Suicidal Inpatients," *Archives of General Psychiatry,* vol. 45, June 1988.

Breslau, Naomi, Davis, Glenn C., and Prabucki, Kenneth, "Searching for Evidence on the Validity of Generalized Anxiety Disorder: Psychopathology in Children of Anxious Mothers," *Psychiatry Research,* no. 20, 1987.

Brody, Jane E., "Trip Across Adolescence Is Just as Risky as Ever," Personal Health column, *The New York Times,* March 3, 1988.

Byrne, Robert, *The Third—and Possibly the Best—637 Best Things Anybody Ever Said.* New York: Atheneum, 1986.

Cadwalader, George, *Castaways: The Penikese Island Experiment,* Chelsea, VT: Chelsea Green Publishing Company, 1988.

Campbell, Magda, M.D., and Spencer, Elizabeth Kay, M.D., "Psychopharmacology in Child and Adolescent Psychiatry: A Review of the Past Five Years," *Journal of the American Academy of Child and Adolescent Psychiatry,* vol. 27, no. 3., 1988.

Cantwell, Dennis P., M.D., and Hanna, Gregory L., M.D., "Attention-Deficit Hyperactivity Disorder," *American Psychiatric Press Review of Psychiatry,* vol. 8, Allan Tasman, M.D., Robert E. Hales, M.D., and Allen J. Frances, M.D., eds. Washington, D.C.: American Psychiatric Press, Inc., 1989.

Carlson, Gabrielle A., M.D., "Bipolar Disorder in Adolescence," *Psychiatric Annals,* vol. 15, no. 6, June 1985.

Carter, Betty, M.S.W., and McGoldrick, Monica, M.S.W., "Overview: The Changing Family Life Cycle: A Framework for Family Therapy," *The Changing Family Life Cycle: A Framework for Family Therapy,* second edition, Betty Carter, M.S.W., and Monica McGoldrick, M.S.W., eds. New York and London: Gardner Press, 1989.

Chagoya, Leopoldo, M.D., and Schkolne, Theo, M.A., "Children Who Lie: A Review of the Literature," *Canadian Journal of Psychiatry,* vol. 31, October 1986.

Chamberlain, P., and Patterson, G. R., "Aggressive Behavior in Middle Childhood," *The Clinical Guide to Psychiatry,* D. Shaffer, ed. New York: The Free Press, 1985.

Chatlos, Calvin, M.D., with Chilnick, Lawrence D., *Crack: What you Should Know About the Cocaine Epidemic.* New York: Perigee Books, 1987.

Chess, Stella, M.D., and Hassibi, Mahin, M.D., *Principles and Practice of Child Psychiatry.* New York and London: Plenum Press, 1978.

Cicchetti, Dante, and Schneider-Rosen, Karen, "Toward a Transactional Model of Childhood Depression," *Childhood Depression,* Dante Cicchetti and Karen Schneider-Rosen, eds. A part of *New Directions for Child Development,* William Damon, editor-in-chief, no. 26, December 1984. San Francisco: Jossey-Bass Inc.

Clark, David C., Ph.D., Gibbons, Robert D., Ph.D., Fawcett, Jan, M.D., and Scheftner, William A., M.D., Young, Michael A., Ph.D., "Predictive Implications of a Suicide Attempt," from the proceedings of the 140th annual meeting of the American Psychiatric Association, 1987.

Cleary, Paul D., Hitchcock, Jan L., Semmer, Norbert, Flinchbaugh, Laura J., and Pinney, John M., "Adolescent Smoking: Research and Health Policy," *The Milbank Quarterly,* vol. 66, no. 1, 1988.

Coble, Patricia A., R.N., Taska, Lynn S., B.A., Kupfer, David J., M.D., Kazdin, Alan E., Ph.D., Unis, Alan, M.D., and French, Nancy, R.N., M.S., "EEG Sleep 'Abnormalities' in Preadolescent Boys with a Diagnosis of Conduct Disorder," *Journal of the American Academy of Child Psychiatry,* vol. 23, no. 4, 1984.

Coddington, R. Dean, "Stress and Its Implications for Child Mental Health," *Basic Handbook of Child Psychiatry,* vol. 5: *Advances and New Directions,* Joseph D. Noshpitz, editor-in-chief, et al. New York: Basic Books, Inc., 1987.

Conners, C. Keith, and Werry, John S., "Pharmacotherapy," *Psychopathological Disorders of Childhood,* second edition, Herbert C. Quay and John S. Werry, eds. New York: John Wiley & Sons, 1972, 1979.

Conroy, Robert W., M.D., "The Many Facets of Adolescent Drinking," *Bulletin of the Menninger Clinic,* no. 52, 1988.

Cytryn, Leon, and McKnew, Donald H., Jr., "Childhood Depression: An Update," *Basic Handbook of Child Psychiatry,* vol. 5: *Advances and New Directions,* Joseph D. Noshpitz, editor-in-chief, et al. New York: Basic Books, Inc., 1987.

———, "Treatment of Childhood Depression," *Basic Handbook of Child Psychiatry,* vol. 5: *Advances and New Directions,* Joseph D. Noshpitz, editor-in-chief, et al. New York: Basic Books, Inc., 1987.

Czechowicz, Dorynne, M.D., "Adolescent Alcohol and Drug Abuse and Its Consequences—An Overview," *American Journal of Drug and Alcohol Abuse,* vol. 14, no. 2, 1988.

Dougherty, Margot, and Di Giovanni, Janine, "Kay Kent Died the Way She Lived—As a Mirror of Marilyn Monroe," *People,* July 3, 1989.

Ebels, Ebel J., "Maturation of the Central Nervous System," *Developmental Psychiatry,* Michael Rutter, ed. Washington, D.C.: American Psychiatric Press, Inc., 1980.

Elliott, Ruth S., with Savage, Jim, *The Complete Practical Guide to Hiring, Training, Living With, and Firing Nannies, Caregivers, Babysitters, Au Pairs.* New York: Prentice-Hall Press, 1990.

Fawcett, Jan, M.D., Scheftner, William, M.D., Fogg, Louis, Ph.D., Clark, David, Ph.D., and Young, Michael, Ph.D., "Acute vs. Long-Term Predictors of Suicide," from the proceedings of the 140th annual meeting of the American Psychiatric Association, 1987.

Felthous, Alan R., M.D., and Kellert, Stephen R., Ph.D., "Childhood Cruelty to Animals and Later Aggression Against People: A Review," *American Journal of Psychiatry,* vol. 144, no. 6, June 1987.

Freeman, Patricia, and Armstrong, Lois, "Actress Marlee Matlin Builds a Bridge to Silence to Star in Her First Speaking Role," *People,* April 10, 1989.

Friedman, Alfred S., Ph.D., Glicksman, Nita W., M.S., M.P.H., and Morrissey, Margaret R., B.S., "What Mothers Know About Their Adolescents' Alcohol/Drug Use and Problems, and How Mothers React to Finding Out About It," *Journal of Drug Education,* vol. 18, no. 2, 1988.

Gardner, Sandra, with Rosenberg, Gary, M.D., *Teenage Suicide.* New York: Julian Messner, 1985.

Ginott, Haim G., *Teacher and Child: A Book for Parents and Teachers.* New York: Avon Books, 1972.

Gittelman, Rachel, Ph.D., "Treatment of Reading Disorders," *Developmental Neuropsychiatry,* Michael Rutter, ed. New York and London: The Guilford Press, 1983.

————, Mannuzza, Salvatore, Ph.D., Shenker, Ronald, M.D., and Bonagura, Noreen, M.S.W., "Hyperactive Boys Almost Grown Up: I. Psychiatric Status," *Archives of General Psychiatry,* vol. 42, October 1985.

Gold, Mark S., M.D., *The Good News About Panic, Anxiety, and Phobias.* New York: Villard Books, 1989.

————, with Morris, Lois B., *The Good News About Depression: Cures and Treatments in the New Age of Psychiatry.* New York: Bantam Books, 1986.

Goleman, Daniel, "Depressed Parents Put Children at a Greater Risk of Depression," *The New York Times,* March 30, 1989.

Gordon, Thomas, *Parental Effectiveness Training (P.E.T.) in Action: The No-Lose Way to Raise Happier, More Responsible, More Cooperative Children.* New York: Bantam Books, 1988.

Gould, Madelyn S., Ph.D., M.P.H., and Shaffer, David, M.D., "The Impact of Suicide in Television Movies: Evidence of Imitation," *The New England Journal of Medicine,* September 11, 1986.

Graham, Philip J., "Epidemiological Studies," *Psychopathological Disorders of Childhood,* second edition, Herbert C. Quay and John S. Werry, eds. New York: John Wiley & Sons, 1972, 1979.

Greenhill, Laurence L., "Pediatric Psychopharmacology," *The Clinical Guide to Child Psychiatry,* David Shaffer et al, eds. New York: The Free Press, 1984.

Gross, David A., M.D., and Extein, Irl L., M.D., *A Parent's Guide to Common and Uncommon School Problems.* Summit, NJ: The PIA Press, 1989.

Hayes, Peter A., D.M.D., M.S., M.R.C.D., Prince, Michael T., Ph.D., and Hayes, Kimberley, "The Suicidal Adolescent," *Journal of Dentistry for Children,* March–April 1987.

Hendren, Robert Lee, D.O., "Adolescent Alcoholism and Substance Abuse," *American Psychiatric Association Annual Review,* vol. 5, Allen J. Frances, M.D. and Robert E. Hales, M.D., eds. Washington, D.C.: American Psychiatric Press, Inc., 1986.

Hetherington, E. Mavis, and Martin, Barclay, "Family Interaction," *Psychopathological Disorders of Childhood,* second edition, Herbert C. Quay and John S. Werry, eds. New York: John Wiley & Sons, 1972, 1979.

Hinde, R. A., "Family Influences," *Developmental Psychiatry,* Michael Rutter, ed. Washington, D.C.: American Psychiatric Press, Inc. 1980.

Hsu, L. K. George, "An Overview of the Eating Disorders," *Basic Handbook of Child Psychiatry,* vol. 5: *Advances and New Directions,* Joseph D. Noshpitz, editor-in-chief, et al. New York: Basic Books, Inc., 1987.

Hunt, Robert D., Brunstetter, Richard W., and Silver, Larry B., "Attention Deficit Disorder: Diagnosis and Etiology," *Basic Handbook of Child Psychiatry,* vol. 5: *Advances and New Directions,* Joseph D. Noshpitz, editor-in-chief, et al. New York: Basic Books, Inc., 1987.

Irwin, Charles E., Jr., and Vaughan, Elaine, "Psychosocial Context of Adolescent Development: Study Group Report," *Journal of Adolescent Health Care,* vol. 9, 1988.

Jensen, Major Peter S., M.D., Bain, Lieutenant Colonel Michael W., M.D., and Josephson, Allen M., M.D., "Why Johnny Can't Sit Still: Kids' Ideas Why They Take Stimulants," presented at the American Psychological Association, San Francisco, May 1989.

Joshi, Paramjit T., M.D., Capozzoli, Joseph A., R.N., and Coyle, Joseph T., M.D., "Use of a Quiet Room on an Inpatient Unit," *Journal of the American Academy of Child and Adolescent Psychiatry,* no. 27, 1988.

Kashani, Javad H., M.D., Anasserile Daniel, E., M.D., Sulzberger, Leigh A., Rosenberg, Tomas K., M.A., and Reid, John C., Ph.D., "Conduct Disordered Adolescents from a Community Sample," *Canadian Journal of Psychiatry,* vol. 32, December 1987.

Kay, Rena L., M.D., and Kay, Jerald, M.D., "Adolescent Conduct Disorders," *American Psychiatric Association Annual Review,* vol. 5, Allen J.

Frances, M.D., and Robert E. Hales, M.D., eds. Washington, D.C.: American Psychiatric Press, Inc., 1986.

Kazdin, Alan E., "Advances in Child Behavior Therapy," *Basic Handbook of Child Psychiatry,* vol. 5: *Advances and New Directions,* Joseph D. Noshpitz, editor-in-chief, et al. New York: Basic Books, Inc., 1987.

Keith, Charles R., "Violent Youth," *Basic Handbook of Child Psychiatry,* vol. 5: *Advances and New Directions,* Joseph D. Noshpitz, editor-in-chief, et al. New York: Basic Books, Inc., 1987.

Kett, Joseph, *Rites of Passage: Adolescents in America 1790 to the Present.* New York: Basic Books, 1977.

Kübler-Ross, Elisabeth, *On Death and Dying,* New York: Macmillan Publishing Co., 1969.

Kutner, Lawrence, "The Stresses and Power Plays of Adolescence," Parent and Child column, *The New York Times,* March 3, 1988.

Leonard, Henrietta L., M.D., and Rapoport, Judith L., M.D., "Anxiety Disorders in Childhood and Adolescence," *American Psychiatric Press Review of Psychiatry,* vol. 8, Allan Tasman, M.D., Robert E. Hales, M.D., and Allen J. Frances, M.D., eds. Washington, D.C.: American Psychiatric Press, Inc. 1989.

Leonard, Henrietta, L., M.D., Swedo, Susan, M.D., Rapoport, Judith L., M.D., Coffey, Marge, M.S.W., and Cheslow, Deborah, B.S., "Treatment of Childhood Obsessive Compulsive Disorder with Clomipramine and Desmethylimipramine: A Double-Blind Crossover Comparison," *Psychopharmacology Bulletin,* vol. 24, no. 1, 1988.

Levin, Eric, "The Fighting, Loving O'Neal Clan," *People,* August 15, 1983.

———, "Picking Up the Pieces," *People,* June 4, 1984.

Levine, Frederick M., and Kathleen M. Anesko, *Winning the Homework War,* New York: Prentice Hall, 1987.

Lewis, Dorothy Otnow, M.D., "Juvenile Delinquency," *The Clinical Guide to Child Psychiatry,* David Shaffer et al, eds. New York: The Free Press, 1984.

———, Lewis, Melvin, M.B.B.S., F.R.C.Psych., D.C.H., Unger, Lisa, and Goldman, Clifford, "Conduct Disorder and Its Synonyms: Diagnoses of Dubious Validity and Usefulness," *American Journal of Psychiatry,* vol. 141, no. 4, April 1984.

McGuinness, Diane, *When Children Don't Learn: Understanding the Biology and Psychology of Learning Disabilities.* New York: Basic Books, Inc., 1985.

Maccoby, Eleanor E., and Jacklin, Carol Nagy, "Psychological Sex Differences," *Developmental Psychiatry,* Michael Rutter, ed. Washington, D.C.: American Psychiatric Press, Inc., 1980.

Mahler, Margaret S., Pine, Fred, and Bergman, Anni, *The Psychological Birth of the Human Infant: Symbiosis and Individuation.* New York: Basic Books, Inc., 1975.

Manning, Anita, "Teens and Sex in the Age of AIDS," *USA Today,* October 3, 1988.

————, "What Kids Want to Know About Sex," Health and Behavior column, *USA Today,* October 3, 1988.

Mannuzza, Salvatore, Ph.D., Klein, Rachel Gittelman, Ph.D., Bonagura, Noreen, M.S.W., Konig, Paula Horowitz, and Shenker, Ronald, M.D., "Hyperactive Boys Almost Grown Up: II. Status of Subjects Without a Mental Disorder," *Archives of General Psychiatry,* vol. 45, January 1988.

Marriage, Keith, MB., F.R.C.P., Fine, Stuart, M.B., F.R.C.P., Moretti, Marlene, M.A., and Haley, Glenn, M.A., "Relationship Between Depression and Conduct Disorder in Children and Adolescents," *Journal of the American Academy of Child Psychiatry,* vol. 25, no. 5, 1986.

Mattison, Richard E., M.D., "Suicide and Other Consequences of Childhood and Adolescent Anxiety Disorders," *Journal of Clinical Psychiatry,* vol. 49, no. 10, October 1988.

Meeks, John E., M.D., *High Times/Low Times: The Many Faces of Adolescent Depression.* Summit, NJ: The PIA Press, 1988.

Melpomene Institute for Women's Health Research, *Bodywise: The Melpomene Guide for Physically Active Women,* New York: Prentice Hall Press, 1990.

Mitchell, James E., "Anorexia Nervosa: Medical and Physiological Aspects," *Handbook of Eating Disorders: Physiology, Psychology, and Treatment of Obesity, Anorexia, and Bulimia,* Kelly D. Brownell and John P. Foreyt, eds. New York: Basic Books, Inc., 1986.

Moyes, Theresa, Tennent, T. Gavin, and Bedford, Anthony P., "Long Term Follow-up Study of a Ward-Based Behaviour Modification Programme for Adolescents with Acting-Out and Conduct Problems," *British Journal of Psychiatry,* no. 147, 1985.

The National Association of Private Psychiatric Hospitals, *Teenagers at Risk: An Adult Perspective,* Washington, D.C.: Press Release Package on Survey, September 12, 1988.

————, *Our Troubled Youth: A Statistical Profile,* Washington, D.C.: Press Release. September 12, 1988.

Neiger, Brad L., and Hopkins, Rodney W., "Adolescent Suicide: Character Traits of High-Risk Teenagers," *Adolescence,* vol. 23, no. 90, Summer 1988.

Newcomb, Michael D., and Bentler, P. M., "Impact of Adolescent Drug Use and Social Support on Problems of Young Adults: A Longitudinal Study," *Journal of Abnormal Psychology,* vol. 97, no. 1, 1988.

Newman, Michael M., M.D., and Rayfield, Gina E., Ph.D., *The Eating Disorders: Anorexia Nervosa, Bulimia Nervosa and Compulsive Overeating.* (pamphlet) Summit, NJ: Fair Oaks Hospital.

Nubel, Aviva S., R.N., M.S., and Solomon, Linda Zener, Ph.D., "Addicted Adolescent Girls: Familial Interpersonal Relationships," *Journal of Psychosocial Nursing,* vol. 26, no. 1, 1988.

Offer, Daniel, Ostrov, Eric, and Howard, Kenneth I., *The Adolescent: A Psychological Self-Portrait.* New York: Basic Books, Inc., 1981.

Ouston, Janet, Maughan, Barbara, and Mortimore, Peter, "School Influences," *Developmental Psychiatry,* ed. by Michael Rutter. Washington, D.C.: American Psychiatric Press, Inc., 1980.

Petti, Theodore A., Benswanger, Ellen G., and Fialkov, M. Jerome, "The Rural Child and Child Psychiatry," *Basic Handbook of Child Psychiatry,* vol. 5: *Advances and New Directions,* Joseph D. Noshpitz, editor-in-chief, et al. New York: Basic Books, Inc., 1987.

Pfeffer, Cynthia R., M.D., "Self-Destructive Behavior in Children and Adolescents," *Psychiatric Clinics of North America,* vol. 8, no. 2, June 1985.

Pfefferbaum, Betty, M.D., "Adolescence and Illness," *American Psychiatric Association Annual Review,* vol. 5, Allen J. Frances, M.D., and Robert E. Hales, M.D., eds. Washington, D.C.: American Psychiatric Press, Inc., 1986.

Plummer, William, "Two Months After the Boating Accident, Griffin O'Neal Is Indicted in the Death of Friend Gio Coppola," *People,* August 11, 1986.

Pomeroy, John C., M.B.B.S., M.R.C., "Periodicity, Pubescence and Psychiatric Disturbance," *Psychiatry Newsletter.* Summit, NJ: Fair Oaks Hospital, Winter 1989.

Preto, Nydia Garcia, A.C.S.W., "Transformation of the Family System in Adolescence," *The Changing Family Life Cycle: A Framework for Family Therapy,* second edition, Betty Carter, M.S.W., and Monica McGoldrick, M.S.W., eds. New York and London: Gardner Press, 1989.

Price, Neil D., M.D., *On the Edge: The Love/Hate World of the Borderline Personality.* Summit, NJ: The PIA Press, 1989.

Rapoport, Judith L., "Congenital Anomalies, Appearance and Body Build," *Developmental Psychiatry,* Michael Rutter, ed. Washington, D.C.: American Psychiatric Press, Inc., 1980.

Reeves, Jan C., M.B.Ch.B., M.R.A.N.Z.C.P., Werry, John S., M.D., Elkind, Gail S., Ph.D., and Zametkin, Alan, M.D., "Attention Deficit, Conduct, Oppositional, and Anxiety Disorders in Children: II. Clinical Characteristics," *Journal of the American Academy of Child and Adolescent Psychiatry,* vol. 26, no. 2, 1987.

Reynolds, Ingrid, and Rob, Marilyn I., "The Role of Family Difficulties in Adolescent Depression, Drug-Taking, and Other Family Problems," *The Medical Journal of Australia,* vol. 149, September 5, 1988.

Rich, Dorothy, *MegaSkills: How Families Can Help Children Succeed in School and Beyond.* Boston: Houghton Mifflin Company, 1988.

Rifkin, Arthur, M.D., Wortman, Richard, M.D., Reardon, Gerard, M.S.W., Siris, Samuel G., "Psychotropic Medication in Adolescents: A Review," *Journal of Clinical Psychiatry,* vol. 47, no. 8, August 1986.

Robins, Lee N., "Follow-up Studies," *Psychopathological Disorders of Childhood,* second edition, Herbert C. Quay and John S. Werry, eds. New York: John Wiley & Sons, 1972, 1979.

Ross, Alan O., and Nelson, Rosemary O., "Behavior Therapy," *Psychopathological Disorders of Childhood,* second edition, Herbert C. Quay and John S. Werry, eds. New York: John Wiley & Sons, 1972, 1979.

Rudolph, Ileane, and Rosenthal, Herma, "Life Goes On: Will Viewers Accept a TV Star with Down Syndrome?" *TV Guide,* July 22, 1989.

Rutter, Michael, "Attachment and the Development of Social Relationships," *Developmental Psychiatry,* Michael Rutter, ed. Washington, DC: American Psychiatric Press, Inc., 1980.

———, *Changing Youth in a Changing Society: Patterns of Adolescent Development and Disorder.* Cambridge, MA: Harvard University Press, 1980.

———, "Psychosexual Development," *Developmental Psychiatry,* Michael Rutter, ed. Washington, D.C.: American Psychiatric Press, Inc., 1980.

———, Chadwick, Oliver, and Shaffer, David, "Head Injury," *Developmental Neuropsychiatry,* Michael Rutter, ed. New York and London: The Guilford Press, 1983.

Ryan, Neal D., M.D., and Puig-Antich, Joaquim, M.D., "Pharmacological Treatment of Adolescent Psychiatric Disorders," *Journal of Adolescent Health Care,* vol. 8, no. 1, January 1987.

Safer, Daniel J., M.D., and Allen, Richard P., Ph.D., "Stimulant Drug Treatment of Hyperactive Adolescents," *Diseases of the Nervous System,* no. 36, 1975.

Satterfield, James H., M.D., Hoppe, Christiane M., Ph.D., and Schell, Anne M., Ph.D., "A Prospective Study of Delinquency in 110 Adolescent Boys with Attention Deficit Disorder and 88 Normal Adolescent Boys," *American Journal of Psychiatry,* vol. 139, no. 6, June 1982.

Scott, Elizabeth S., and Derdeyn, Andre P., "Children and the Law: The Psychiatrist as Court Consultant," *Basic Handbook of Child Psychiatry,* vol. 5: *Advances and New Directions,* Joseph D. Noshpitz, editor-in-chief, et al. New York: Basic Books, Inc., 1987.

Shaffer, David, M.B., F.R.C.P., F.R.C.Psych, "The Epidemiology of Teen Suicide: An Examination of Risk Factors," *Journal of Clinical Psychiatry,* vol. 49, no. 9, September 1988.

———, "Suicide in Childhood and Early Adolescence," *Journal of Child Psychology and Psychiatry,* vol. 15, 1974.

Shields, James, "Genetics and Mental Development," *Developmental Psychiatry,* Michael Rutter, ed. Washington, D.C.: American Psychiatric Press, Inc., 1980.

Silver, Larry B., and Brunstetter, Richard W., "Learning Disabilities: Recent Advances," *Basic Handbook of Child Psychiatry,* vol. 5: *Advances and New Directions,* Joseph D. Noshpitz, editor-in-chief, et al. New York: Basic Books, Inc., 1987.

Slaby, Andrew E., M.D., Ph.D., M.P.H., *Aftershock: Surviving the Delayed Effects of Trauma, Crisis and Loss.* New York: Villard Books, 1989.

Steinman, Susan B., D.S.W., Zemmelman, Steven E., M.S.W., and Knoblauch, Thomas M., Ph.D., "A Study of Parents Who Sought Joint Custody Following Divorce: Who Reaches Agreement and Sustains Joint Custody and Who Returns to Court," *Journal of the American Academy of Child Psychiatry,* vol. 24, no. 5, 1985.

Strober, Michael, "Anorexia Nervosa: History and Psychological Concepts," *Handbook of Eating Disorders: Physiology, Psychology, and Treatment of Obesity, Anorexia, and Bulimia,* Kelly D. Brownell and John P. Foreyt, eds. New York: Basic Books, Inc., 1986.

Tanguay, Peter E., "Cognition and Psychopathology," *Basic Handbook of Child Psychiatry,* vol. 5: *Advances and New Directions,* Joseph D. Noshpitz, editor-in-chief, et al. New York: Basic Books, Inc., 1987.

Thorley, G., "Adolescent Outcome for Hyperactive Children," *Archives of Disease in Childhood,* vol. 63, 1988.

Trautman, P.D., M.D., and Rotheram-Borus, M.J., Ph.D., "Cognitive Behavior Therapy with Children and Adolescents," in *American Psychiatric Press Review of Psychiatry,* vol. 7, ed. by Frances, A. J., and Hales, R. E. Washington, D.C.: American Psychiatric Press, Inc., 1988.

Walker, Jason L., Lahey, Benjamin B., Hynd, George W., and Frame, Cynthia L., "Comparison of Specific Patterns of Antisocial Behavior in Children with Conduct Disorder With or Without Coexisting Hyperactivity," *Journal of Consulting and Clinical Psychology,* vol. 55, no. 6, 1987.

Webster-Stratton, Carolyn, "Comparison of Abusive and Nonabusive Families with Conduct-Disordered Children," *American Journal of Orthopsychiatry,* vol. 55, no. 1, January 1985.

————, "Randomized Trial of Two Parent-Training Programs for Families with Conduct-Disordered Children," *Journal of Consulting and Clinical Psychology,* vol. 52, no. 4, 1984.

Weiner, Barbara A., J.D., "An Overview of Child Custody Laws," *Hospital and Community Psychiatry,* vol. 36, no. 8, August 1985.

Weisberg, Lynne W., M.D., Ph.D., and Greenberg, Rosalie, M.D., *When Acting Out Isn't Acting Out: Understanding Child and Adolescent Temper, Anger and Behavior Disorders.* Summit, NJ: The PIA Press, 1988.

Weiss, Gabrielle, M.D., Hechtman, Lily, M.D., Milroy, Thomas, M.D., and Perlman, Terrye, M.S., "Psychiatric Status of Hyperactives as Adults: A Controlled Prospective 15-Year Follow-up of 63 Hyperactive Children," *Journal of the American Academy of Child Psychiatry,* vol. 24, no. 2, 1985.

Werry, John S., M.D., Reeves, Jan Catherine, M.B. Ch.B., M.R.A.N.Z.C.P., and Elkind, Gail S., Ph.D., "Attention Deficit, Conduct, Oppositional, and Anxiety Disorders in Children: I. A Review of Research on Differentiating Characteristics," *Journal of American Academy of Child and Adolescent Psychiatry,* vol. 26, no. 2, 1987.

Yalom, Irvin D., "Breaking Silence: Glamour Readers Talk About Childhood Sexual Abuse, and How It Changed Their Lives," *Glamour,* June 1989.

————, "Day Care Dilemma Leaves Parents Pressured, Confused," *Psychiatric News,* January 1989.

————, *Diagnostic and Statistical Manual of Mental Disorders,* third edition, revised. Washington, DC: American Psychiatric Association, 1987.

————, "Georgia Teen-Age Suicides Studied," *The New York Times,* October 26, 1988.

————, "Maryland Jury Indicts O'Neal for Manslaughter in Coppola Son's Death," *Variety,* July 30, 1986.

————, "Selection of Subjects for Study of Depression in Adolescents," Letters to the Editor, *American Journal of Psychiatry,* vol. 145, no. 3, March 1988.

————, *The Theory and Practice of Group Psychotherapy,* third edition. New York: Basic Books, Inc., 1988.

INDEX

ABOUT THE AUTHOR

LARRY E. DUMONT, M.D., is director of the Adolescent Treatment Unit at Fair Oaks Hospital. Dr. Dumont received his B.A. from Tulane University and his M.D. from Northwestern University School of Medicine. After his internship and adult psychiatry residency at Tulane, he completed his child and adolescent fellowship at New York University. He is a member of the American Academy of Child Psychiatry, and he teaches and lectures on adolescent depression. Dr. Dumont is the author of *A Parent's Guide to Teens and Cults,* as well as several other publications.